the INside

the INside effects

How the Body Heals Itself

Featuring:

Dr. John Demartini, Lynne McTaggart, and JP Sears

— and —

Contributing Authors – Regina Altamirano, Melissa Deally,
Sally Estlin, Dr. Karen Kan G, Mark Hattas, PhD (h.c.),
Patra Healey, Cathy Hohmeyer, Cheri Lowman, Sylvie Olivier,
Shannon Procise, Keith Leon S., Maura Leon S.,
Trisha Schmalhofer, Sharla Lee Shults,
Dr. Elizabeth Hesse Sheehan, Dr. Odette Suter,
Nicole Thibodeau, Marie-Laure Will, and Dr. Liz Winders

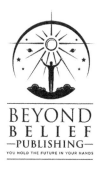

BEYOND
BELIEF
—PUBLISHING—
YOU HOLD THE FUTURE IN YOUR HANDS

ISBN: 978-1-957972-13-8

This book was created in honor of all the practitioners dedicated to natural healing and all who are committed to healing themselves naturally.

Contents

Acknowledgments

It is with deep appreciation that I thank all the authors who said yes to participating in *the INside effects* film project: Darius Barazandeh, Marcus Bird, Kathleen Bobak, Lee Carroll, Kyle Cease, Deanna Courtney, Tom Cowan, Dr. John Demartini, Kim D'Eramo, Julie Renee Doering, Jeffrey Gignac, Mia Hohl, Dr. Karen Kan G, Andrew Kaufman, Dr. Cathleen King, Erin Kinney, Matty Lansdown, MariaElena Marks, Rollin McCraty, Lynne McTaggart, Monika Muranyi, Bradley Nelson, Clint G. Rogers, Ken Rohla, JP Sears, Craig Shoemaker, Amandha Vollmer, Lisa Warner, and Mikki Willis.

Thank you to Erik Arthur Peterson, Theo Hall, Jordan Craig, Brian Dillon, Gabriel Valda, Callum Shallenberger, Mikal Masters, Nevaeh Pillsbury, Cruz Christian Carriere, Drew Thomsen, Erik Van Yserloo, Bob Sima, Shannon Plummer, Trisha Schmalhofer, and Maura Leon S. for your participation during the film-making process and after.

Thanks to Bob Proctor, Jack Canfield, Adam Markel, Joe Vitale, Michael Beckwith, Rickie Byars, and John Demartini for being such great mentors and for always saying yes. Your support over the years has been instrumental in my success as an author, publisher, and now a filmmaker.

Thank you to our incredible team who brought this book forward to completion and to the world one step at a time: Maggie Mills, Heather Taylor, Bethany Knowles, Autumn Carlton, Maryna Zhukova, and Rudy Milanovich.

Introduction

When we decided to start a publishing business twenty years ago, we were very clear about the authors we wanted to publish. Our mentors had taught us "You are the five people you spend the most time with." We wanted to surround ourselves with successful, cutting-edge difference-makers. Because of this, the first fifty books we published were authored by functional medicine doctors. Functional medicine doctors are *medical professionals who specialize in finding the root causes of disease.* They work holistically, considering the full picture of your physical, emotional, mental, and sometimes even spiritual health, considering factors like diet, hormonal changes, genetics, prescription and over-the-counter medications, and other lifestyle choices.

We soon discovered the people we wanted to serve the most were so busy being in service to others that they didn't have time to sit down and write a book themselves. They needed a book to share about their mission, their vision, and their gifts, but had no time to write it. This led us to the creation of a process we call The YouSpeakIt Book Program.

Our process allows difference-makers to attend seven phone calls. In those seven calls, we lead them through speaking their book. The YouSpeakIt process brings ease and grace to the creation of a book, and this process is one of the qualities that sets us apart from other publishers.

While working with these medical professionals and reading their books, we learned a lot about the body's ability to heal itself. Keith had an experience as a child when his aunt used nontraditional healing methods, and her cancer dissolved and disappeared in two weeks. This implanted into his mind the thought and belief: The body has the ability to heal itself, which is why he decided that for his first full-feature film, he would produce and direct a documentary called *the INside effects: How the Body Heals Itself.* Creating this film has allowed him to dive into the subject he has such a passion for. This film, and the doctors, scientists, and health advocates he interviewed, not only validated many of his beliefs but opened a new world of information that he hadn't studied and researched.

Keith realized at one point during production that he would be able to interview only a certain number of experts, and the questions he was asking each health advocate in the film covered three main topics. He thought: I want to provide people who have just watched the film with their next steps and introduce them to more experts. This is when the idea for this book was born. Its focus is on one thing and one thing alone: now that you have learned that the body does indeed have the ability to heal, how do you support it to do so?

We have purposely asked each expert the same three questions. This allows you to receive specific answers regarding healing while allowing you to feel into who are the best teachers for you. We suggest you reach out to those you feel most connected to, work with them, and hire them. If you've discovered this book without seeing the movie, we highly suggest you watch it (theINsideeffects.com), as the film is also created to introduce you to the top experts in their field. Reach out to them as well.

We trust this book will guide you to learning and discovering alternative methods for healing. It has been an absolute pleasure to interview the authors and provide this valuable information. Enjoy the read.

Warmly,

Keith and Maura Leon S.

BeyondBeliefPublishing.com
LeonSmithPublishing.com
YouSpeakItBooks.com
BabypiePublishing.com

Regina Altamirano

WHEN AND HOW DID YOU FIRST DISCOVER THE BODY HAS THE INNATE ABILITY TO HEAL ITSELF?

In 1968, when I was eleven, my mother started having severe headaches. Doctors found a tumor in her brain that grew around her pituitary gland. It was nonmalignant, but, unfortunately, the tumor kept returning, and she endured eight brain surgeries over the next ten years.

About once every year, surgery was necessary to remove a newly developed tumor, and I witnessed her body heal every time. Still, I couldn't understand why these tumors were happening again and again. So, I began reading, researching, and watching videos about the brain, the body, and healing.

Due to complications, the last three surgeries were done consecutively within less than a month. At that time, doctors didn't know the vital functions of the pituitary gland, so they removed it. Without going into detail, I can honestly say the procedures after that were no less than barbaric. The person I knew as my beautiful mother could no longer see, walk, or control bodily functions.

Because of the emotional and physical pain that my mother and entire family endured, I developed a distrust of doctors. Consequently, I began a lifelong quest to discover the *how* of the body's innate ability to heal itself. As a result, I became a dedicated student of psychology, anatomy, movement, metaphysics, essential oils, and subtle energy.

In 2014, my then-boyfriend had a stroke one morning while getting dressed. When I saw what was happening, I immediately called the paramedics and went into action using the tools and techniques I had learned and practiced over the years. I visualized him, and the paramedics, doctors, nurses, and technicians who would treat him, surrounded in white light while I prayed and drove to the hospital.

In the emergency room, while we awaited testing, his heart stopped, and he had to be resuscitated. Then, after several tests, the doctors told me he had suffered a bilateral stroke and paralysis on the left side.

I asked to have a cot brought to his room for me to sleep on. Throughout the night, whenever he would move or make a sound, I would do energy work on him and run a LifeLine treatment, which is an integrative therapeutic system that assists in processing emotions buried in the subconscious mind. When the physical therapist, cardiologist, and neurologist came the next day to assess him, there was no paralysis. Four days and several tests after being admitted, he could go home.

Over the years, I have witnessed what many would call *miracles*. As a result, I deeply respect and appreciate the mind-body-spirit connection and know, without a doubt, that the body has an innate ability to heal.

WHY DO YOU THINK IT'S SO IMPORTANT FOR PEOPLE TO BE AWARE OF HOW THE BODY HEALS ITSELF?

I believe it is crucial to be aware of how the body heals itself so each person can support the process. In addition, knowing it is in the body's DNA blueprint to heal, regenerate, and thrive helps one relax during the healing process and stay out of fear. The more one understands how the body, the mind, and the spirit interact in symbiosis, the faster the healing.

One of the most powerful tools for healing the body is innate within every one of us—that is, the mind. The mind can bring about miraculous outcomes concerning one's health and well-being.

Take, for instance, the placebo effect. Several studies have established that placebo effects result from the power of suggestion and the brain's role in physical health. Imagination is a powerful mind resource and can play a significant role in healing. No matter your current circumstances, if you can imagine something better for yourself, you can create it. Simply stated, the power of imagination, visualization, and belief is quite magical.

Also, being aware that the words you choose have a tremendous impact—whether verbal, written, or in thought form—is vitally important. The saying *sticks and stones will break my bones, but words will never harm me* is a big fat lie. You will never speak to anyone more than you talk to yourself, especially in your head. Thoughts and words are the programs that run your body and your life. Therefore, how you express yourself and your language affects your well-being.

In reality, you cannot affect one aspect of the self without affecting all. So, the potential for complete healing occurs when one becomes aware of how the body heals. And, when one becomes self-realized, healing becomes imminent.

WHAT ADVICE DO YOU HAVE FOR CREATING HEALTH AND VITALITY FROM THE INSIDE OUT?

The pace of life and change is quickening, so be flexible and open. If you feel nervous, anxious, or upset, stop and take a few deep belly breaths to help ground you. We can live without food and water for days, but we can live without oxygen for only minutes. So pay attention to your body. Fully inhaling and exhaling is a beautiful act of self-love, and you can do it anywhere, anytime, and it will significantly impact your well-being.

Become more aware of how the power of your thoughts directly impacts your life quality. Be mindful of the words you use, especially your self-talk.

Engage in rituals of healthy living—eating clean, exercising, having quality social time, and clearing the mind of minutiae. While these activities are positive interventions in their own right, the level of attention you give them can enhance their benefits.

Connecting with spirit and looking deep into nature can inspire, inform, and ground, nurturing your entire being. Taking time to do this allows the body to relax, frees the mind of chatter, and creates space to receive guidance from Source.

The attention, love, and emotional support you need to give yourself can sometimes be challenging. Still, it can help you feel more comfortable, which can go a long way in healing.

And last but not least, don't hesitate to ask for help.

About the Author

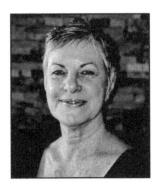

Regina Altamirano is a master-in-training, healer, intuitive coach, and activator. She helps people connect the dots for Self-realization and Self-healing and is passionate about assisting others in harmonizing and healing their body, their life, their relationships, and their environment.

As a teenager, Regina made it her mission to find an answer to the question: *If Jesus said we can do everything he can do and more, then what, exactly, did he do, and how do we do it?* Alas, the quest to find the answer awakened the proverbial seeker and perpetual student. So, joyfully, she is still learning.

Regina's hunger for understanding made her a voracious reader and seeker of knowledge. She focused her studies on psychology, religion, spirituality, and healing arts. Consequently, she is certified in numerous healing modalities and spiritual counseling and holds a bachelor's degree in Metaphysics.

Regina began her private healing practice more than three decades ago. She eventually wound up at Orange County Wellness Center in Southern California under the four-year tutelage of Dr. Ron Jones to practice subtle energy healing and remote viewing.

Shortly after that, Regina assisted Dr. Darren Weissman, founder of LifeLine Technique, for three and a half years at Hay House, *I Can Do It!* conferences. She also facilitated training in several states, teaching people from the United States and other countries the LifeLine Technique and muscle testing.

Today, Regina's continued studies include Tolpakan healing, Dimensional Therapy, and Aboukra Energetics, while working with clients remotely, via Zoom and on the phone.

Regina lives in Indiana with her husband and two Chiweenie fur babies. She loves to read, go on walks, take photographs, and travel.

She'd love to assist you on your unique health and healing journey.

To schedule a free thirty-minute one-on-one discovery call and assessment with Regina, go to: https://calendly.com/healer-coach/discovery-call or visit www.Healer-Coach.com.

Melissa Deally

WHEN AND HOW DID YOU FIRST DISCOVER THE BODY HAS THE INNATE ABILITY TO HEAL ITSELF?

I was in the corporate world, busy building my career, being a wife, and raising our two daughters. Suddenly, I was laid off after twenty-four years without a word of thanks when a much larger corporation bought out my employer. In that moment, I knew three things:

- I would never work for someone else again.

- Whatever I did next had to be more of service to the planet and humanity.

- I had no idea what that would be; however, I was open to being guided.

The next year, I was guided into health and wellness when both my daughters had concussions. Because I wasn't working full time, I was available to closely support their healing journey. I was invited to work at a new holistic clinic to support others in their concussion journey; however, I couldn't get practitioner insurance, as I didn't have any certifications, so this drove me back to school. I began training to become a Health Coach. From the moment I started, I had several ah-ha moments:

- I asked myself: *How is it that I'm in my forties and don't know any of this information about my own body?* If I don't, I'm sure there are many others who don't know either, and I can bring this information to them.

- The science of epigenetics is empowering, as it means we are not a victim of our genetics; rather, we are empowered by our ability to create an environment inside our body that is inhospitable to dis-ease when we know how. This is what I now teach.

- We need to look at the body as a whole, not as its individual parts, because the parts of our body are all interconnected.

I already knew our bones could heal, but I hadn't realized that we can heal our bodies from any dis-ease when we create the right environment. When we support deficiencies (lack of minerals and vitamins), and the toxicities in our physical, mental, emotional, and spiritual body — and release them — we can bring the body back into balance, at which point it will heal itself. Our body is designed to self-heal when we create the environment for it to do so.

WHY DO YOU THINK IT IS SO IMPORTANT FOR PEOPLE TO BE AWARE OF HOW THE BODY HEALS ITSELF?

Your health is your greatest asset; after all, without it, what do you have? You can't build your business or career, raise your family, or live life fully from your sick bed. Yet we've been raised in a culture where we aren't taught how to be proactive in our health, so we do nothing until we get sick. Then we go to the doctor expecting them to make us better.

It is not the doctor's responsibility to make you better; it is your responsibility to look after your health. When you know that your body heals itself, you can be empowered in your health journey as I am today. Your health is a lifelong journey. Knowing how to stay healthy and take responsibility for your health allows you to be in the driver's seat of your greatest asset.

Symptoms are your body's way of talking to you, letting you know there are imbalances and asking you to do something differently. Symptoms are like the engine light in your car — a gentle whisper to get you to take notice. Symptoms should make you curious and prompt you to ask yourself, *Why do I have this symptom?* Then you can start getting to the root cause.

Symptoms aren't to be ignored and labeled as *aging* or *genetics* or *seasonal allergies*. However, this is exactly what society teaches us. We believe that, as we age, we should have pain and less energy, and we accept these conditions as normal and keep on pushing through. Soon your body responds with a bigger symptom, the proverbial two-by-four to slow you down, and if you still push through, watch out for the wrecking ball that lands you in a hospital bed for a while. That is your body's way of ensuring it gets what it needs — rest and time to heal.

Unfortunately, the medical system we have today is a "sick care" business that is more interested in optimizing shareholder profit than optimizing your health. They don't teach prevention; they have no diagnostics for early warning signs and do not look for toxicities and imbalances in the body like we do on the holistic side. Their diagnostics are for diagnosing disease, at which point they will prescribe a drug or surgery or both. Therefore, they can't do much to help you until you are really sick. If you aren't sick enough, you'll be sent away, after being told "it's all in your head, or "there is nothing wrong with you," or "come back if it gets worse."

When you understand that the body can heal itself, you aren't reliant on that system. Instead, you can choose to be empowered in your health, work with a practitioner that can guide you in your journey to optimize your health, and find the imbalances early on when it's far easier to bring the body back into balance. You then have this knowledge for life and can make better choices in living a healthy lifestyle.

Our acute care system is excellent, and I'm grateful for it; however, I choose to take responsibility for my own health so that I don't end up another statistic. Six out of ten Americans have a chronic illness; four in ten have more than one. Even worse, the average North American will spend the last ten years of their life in a nursing home, slowly dying. What could you do if you had those ten years back? End-of-life care is also cost-prohibitive, at $108,000 a year and expected to be $140,000 per year by 2030! That doesn't even cover your medical costs!

Knowing that your body can heal itself, when you create the environment for it to do so, allows you to make different choices and therefore have different outcomes. This is why I love my work; I help people take back their power — the power to live life fully, right to the end. Understanding your body's ability to heal also allows you to get out of the fear trance — the fear of contracting COVID, cancer, Alzheimer's, or dementia, the treatments for which take a heavy toll on your body, relationships, and finances. Knowledge is power and knowing where to turn for support eliminates your fear.

Mindset is critical too. If you don't believe you can heal, you won't — that is the power of your unconscious mind; it will give you exactly what you are focusing on. The mind also doesn't process negatives, so if you are saying to yourself, *I don't want to be sick*, it hears, *I want to be sick*, and gives you more of that.

If you believe you can heal, you will. It is as simple as that. However, your belief must be strong. It must be your priority. Working with a practitioner who also believes you can heal is important. Trying to heal on your own is much harder, partially because it's stressful.

And guess what? The body doesn't heal in a stressed-out state. Accepting the guidance of a practitioner and allowing yourself to relax into the healing journey is the best path to healing. Choose a practitioner who will be with you throughout your journey, not for just one appointment. Your healing journey will not be served if the practitioner tells you briefly what to do, then sends you on your way.

WHAT ADVICE DO YOU HAVE FOR CREATING HEALTH AND VITALITY FROM THE INSIDE OUT?

In today's world, it is critical to detox the physical, mental, emotional, and spiritual bodies. By the time symptoms show up in your physical body, they have already moved through your mental, emotional, and spiritual bodies. If you only clear your physical body of toxins, you can end up right back where you were in a year, due to the toxicity in the other bodies. When you clear all the bodies, and continue a practice of regular detoxing, you truly can create an environment that is *in-hospitable* to disease.

I use functional medicine detoxes to support the physical body. I also use Time Line Therapy® (TLT) to clear the toxins from my other bodies, such as negative emotions and limiting beliefs, which are mental toxins. TLT applies a therapeutic process to the fact that we store our memories in a linear manner in our internal memory storage system. You may not even be aware of these toxins, which can be buried deeply in your unconscious mind—going back to childhood or past generations or past lifetimes—yet they are keeping you stuck or causing *dis-ease*.

After clearing the toxins in all the bodies, you can use hypnotherapy to create the outcomes you want, such as:

- Healing, ten times faster

- Building a strong immune system

- Attaining your ideal weight

- Changing your habits, such as quitting smoking or vaping

- Giving up trigger foods you know are unhealthy for you, yet you eat on a regular basis

If you are trying to create new healthy habits for yourself, you want to use the power of your unconscious mind, as it's fast and effective and can be used in so many ways to improve your health and life with ten thousand times the focus. If you are trying to use willpower to change habits, you are relying solely on your conscious mind, and we know that doesn't work, since eighty percent of people have given up on their New Year's resolutions by the end of January. Your conscious mind only makes up ten percent of your mind, and your unconscious mind makes up the other ninety percent, and it contains the blueprint for your perfect health — yet you haven't been taught the tools to access this. And we know that all learning, all behavior, and all change is unconscious. If you are trying to do it consciously, you are using the wrong part of your mind and the wrong tools, which is hard!

Wouldn't you rather do it the easy way? With hypnotherapy, you are using both minds together and can access all one hundred percent. That is the easy way! Chronic illness and spending ten years in a nursing home is living life the hard, no-fun way! Choose instead to be empowered in your health. Your body is your greatest asset and, unlike your car or your house — your other two big assets — you cannot buy a new body! The wonderful thing about your body is that it is *never* too late to start looking after it. Book a complimentary call with Melissa to start mapping out your healing journey at yourguidedhealthjourney.com.

About the Author

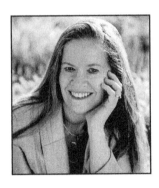

Melissa Deally is your friendly toxin slayer, aka Integrative Mind Body Health Practitioner, also trained in Neurolinguistic Programming and Time Line Therapy, and she is a Hypnotherapy teacher. She's dedicated to helping her clients discover the root cause of their health issue and truly heal, while detoxing their physical, mental, and emotional bodies. Melissa's business is 100 percent virtual.

Melissa uses functional medicine labs mailed to your home while offering a high level of support to ensure your success and achieve lasting results.

Melissa is an international speaker, the winner of the Quality Care Award by Businesses from The Heart in both 2021 and 2022, and she has been named to the 2022 CREA Global Award list. Melissa is the host of the *Don't Wait for Your Wake Up Call!* podcast, offering practical health education, which ranked in the top five percent of Global podcasts in the first three months of launching.

When not serving her clients, Melissa can be found paddleboarding, backcountry hiking and camping with her daughters, and downhill or cross-country skiing. She also devotes time to working on her passion project, Girls Matter, helping to keep girls in school in Uganda, breaking the poverty cycle, one girl, one family, one village at a time.

What are your symptoms trying to tell you? Take Melissa's "Discover Your Toxic Load" quiz here:

bit.ly/mytoxicload

Connect with Melissa and learn more about her programs here:

linktr.ee/yourguidedhealthjourney

Dr. John Demartini

WHEN AND HOW DID YOU FIRST DISCOVER THE BODY HAS THE INNATE ABILITY TO HEAL ITSELF?

I first discovered the body's ability to heal itself when I was seventeen, going on eighteen years old, when I nearly died of strychnine and cyanide poisoning. One night, one hour, one message from one man shifted my perspective, shifted my expectation, shifted the way I saw life, and I saw a transformation in my physiology that I could not ignore. I thought *The power that made the body has the power to heal the body*. I wanted to know the keys and elements that allow people to have the power within to transform their life. They have the power to create the illness. They have the power to transform the illness. Multiple times since then I've had the opportunity to watch clients transform. When they had a transformation on the inside in their psychology, they had a transformation on the outside in their physiology. It is absolutely inspiring to witness, and I've been on this mission for fifty years now because of what I have experienced and witnessed.

WHY DO YOU THINK IT'S SO IMPORTANT FOR PEOPLE TO BE AWARE OF HOW THE BODY HEALS ITSELF?

If you give your power away to other people, their intentions sometimes conflict with your primary intentions. People will overpower you in any area of your life you don't empower. If you don't empower yourself intellectually, you'll be told what to think. If you don't empower your business, you'll be told what to do. If you don't empower finances, you'll be told what you're worth. If you don't empower your relationships, you'll fill your time with "honey do" things that are not inspiring. If you don't empower yourself socially, you'll be told propaganda and misinformation. If you don't empower yourself physically, you'll be told what drugs to take and what organs to remove. If you don't empower yourself spiritually, you'll probably be taught some antiquated dogma. If you don't take command of your life, other people will, and their intentions may not be yours.

It is essential to realize the power you have within and give yourself permission to empower your life and take command of your life when it comes to the healing process and the healing of all areas of your life. If you want to master your life, and not be a victim of history, it is wise to be a master of your destiny.

WHAT ADVICE DO YOU HAVE FOR CREATING HEALTH AND VITALITY FROM THE INSIDE OUT?

Prioritize your life and do not let the outside world dictate your destiny. Make sure the voice and the vision inside of you is louder than all opinions on the outside. Be authentic and true to yourself. If you are trying to be somebody that you're not, you're going to be second at being somebody else, instead of first at being you. Nobody is going to be dedicated to your fulfillment. If you're trying to fit into the world around you, instead of standing out and impacting the world around you, you're going to hold yourself and your physiology back from shining, and you're going to hold yourself back from having vitality.

Your vitality is directly proportionate to the vividness of your vision, the ability to articulate congruently what it is that you feel you are called to do in the world, and your willingness to act according to your own priorities. When you do not give other people permission to encourage you to live by your lower values, you will be liberated to live your life according to your inspiration or higher values.

Do not live to eat; instead, eat to live. Eat to perform. Put high-priority food and fuel into your body so you can live with high and intense vitality. Surround yourself with a high-priority environment that you select. Spend your time, your energy, your money, every aspect of your life on the priorities that are deeply meaningful to you, that allow you to be of service to the world in a sustainable way, in fair exchange, and you will be fulfilled.

Love and gratitude are the two greatest healers. If you do what you love and are grateful for your life, you will have the power to heal from within. Every individual deserves to have the ability to heal themselves. Fill your body with quality water, fresh air, a bit of sunshine, and inspirational knowledge. Surround yourself with people who are inspired by what they do. Prioritize your life, and take command of how you would love to live your life instead of just being a byproduct of the average and the ordinary. Give yourself permission to do something extraordinary. Give yourself permission to have an amazing, inspired, wellness-oriented, and vital life by doing something that's truly meaningful to you.

The difference between us and the animals is that we have the capacity to live with meaning, and doing something meaningful gives us the power to bring order and organization to our physiology. Anytime you're highly infatuated, or highly resentful, or highly emotive, or highly distracted by emotions of the amygdala in the brain, you're robbing yourself of the power and potential to take command of and master your life.

Mastery from within is the same as bringing masterful order into the body; the second you're living by a deeply meaningful, prioritized, and inspired mission, your physiology will help you. Every symptom of your body, every symptom in your psychology, every symptom of your business, every symptom in your social life and in your relationships are feedback mechanisms guiding you to live the true authentic you, the inspired life you deserve, and that is what heals.

You have the capacity to heal yourself. I've seen miraculous transformations. We just had a new case the other day where an individual had leukemia. When they started to go through a complete transformation and prioritization, their life changed. The doctors said, "We must have misdiagnosed it. It's not possible that you had a healing in only weeks." But that individual did. It wasn't a misdiagnosis; the data is there that they transformed from within. The inside effect transformed their life and changed their physiology. This was inspiring. It brings tears to my eyes when I get to see these things repeatedly. You don't frequently hear about it in the news. You don't frequently hear about it at the doctor's office. The truth is you have the power to heal from within. Give yourself permission to release that power by allowing and acknowledging the inside effect.

About the Author

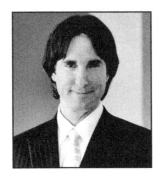

Dr. John Demartini is a polymath and a world-renowned human behavior expert. His work has been described by students as the "most comprehensive body of work" and "an extensive library of wisdom." His mission is to share knowledge and wisdom that empowers you to become a master of your own life and destiny. Dr. D. is an internationally bestselling author, a global educator, and the founder of the Demartini Method, a revolutionary tool in modern psychology. His education curriculum ranges from personal growth seminars to corporate empowerment programs. His teachings are the synthesis of knowledge and wisdom from the greatest minds through history, and his curriculum is designed to help you empower and inspire all areas of your life. Dr. Demartini is the author of over forty-five self-development books and manuscripts, such as the bestseller *The Breakthrough Experience*, which has been translated into dozens of languages. He has produced hundreds of audio and video online courses and products covering subjects such as Building Wealth, Mind-Body Connection, Accessing Your 7 Greatest Powers, Conscious Intention, Powerful Business Insights, and many more. Find out more about products and online learning modules at drdemartini.com

Sally Estlin

WHEN AND HOW DID YOU FIRST DISCOVER THE BODY HAS THE INNATE ABILITY TO HEAL ITSELF?

I was twenty-eight when I had my first real health scare. I was working and partying hard, making great money in banking, and having a lot of laughs. I was oblivious to any real health concerns. I was young and I was having fun!

This was during the 80s and 90s. I thought I was pretty healthy because I was going to the gym every day and had a personal trainer. Banking back then was very much about working hard and playing hard, and my exercise seemed to balance out my work and lifestyle.

It was in the late nineties; I was married at the time and had just relocated to Sydney from Melbourne when I found out I was pregnant.

Wow, that wasn't planned, but I thought *Oh well, it is what it is*. So I went to the docs and was given the usual tests, including an ultrasound and a Pap smear, which I hadn't had for years.

That's when I found out that I had CIN 3—abnormal cells on the surface of the cervix. It's the last stage before cervical cancer if not treated.

I also had a molar pregnancy or a hydatidiform mole, which is a non-cancerous tumor that develops in the uterus due to a nonviable pregnancy.

That was a bit of an eye opener. *Wow, is this for real?* The doctor recommended I have a bit of my cervix burnt off to stop the spread of the cells and a dilation and curettage (DnC) to remove the tumor.

My sister suggested I get a second opinion, so I saw a naturopath. Ultimately, I decided to have the medical procedures; however, that is when I embarked on my own discovery journey and started to understand the amazing ability of our bodies to heal themselves. I was also starting to gain a greater understanding of how illness begins in the body.

I continued to work in banking, but my interest was piqued in natural therapies. For many years I took herbs and homoeopathic remedies and found a lot of ailments like bad allergies and asthma started to clear up. The list started to grow, and I began to feel so much better inside and out.

When I got into yoga, I started to understand that I could find a deeper connection within myself. In addition to just taking drops and herbs and being mindful of our diet and exercise, I was discovering there's a deeper power within us.

Then my mission started. I wanted to understand more about our bodies and how they worked and what helps them heal. I slowly transitioned out of banking and started following my quest for knowledge and understanding. I had two more miscarriages and became insatiable for answers.

I studied aromatherapy and Bach flower remedies to get into the healing power of oils and essences. Then I studied remedial massage and therapies to understand how touch can improve our health and well-being. That led into the study of naturopathy and homeopathy to find the root causes of illness. Then I immersed myself into understanding the power of our guts and how gut health is pivotal to our well-being. Finally, I was drawn into using energy and the quantum field to speed up healing and create health stability.

Of course, nutrition, exercise, and lifestyle are important components that help our bodies heal, but I became fascinated with the power we have within ourselves that uses our own energy to facilitate healing — how our thoughts, feelings, and emotions can powerfully affect us.

Once I truly understood that everything is energy, bigger doors opened to my understanding of our body's ability to step into wellness or illness.

We control our energy, and we can focus our energy to assist our bodies to heal. After all, *Where our attention goes, our energy flows.*

A few years ago, I was given a gardenia bush for my fiftieth birthday. It was healthy and full of divine-smelling buds. As the years went past, it was shoved outside with other potted plants and had withered down to brown sticks with barely any leaves and definitely no flowers.

One of my friends said, "You'll have to throw that out," and I thought *No way. I love that plant.* So for one week, I went outside every day and spoke to that gardenia. I told it I loved it and it could come back to being healthy and vibrant again.

No joke, in just over a week, it started showing green shoots and before long turned into a flourishing bush again.

Wow! If I can focus my energy on a plant, imagine what we could do if we focused positive energy on ourselves. Our bodies have the most amazing ability to react to our emotions and feelings, which are of course energy. We can literally *think ourselves* into wellness or illness.

I dove into the work of Louise Hay and Inna Segal to understand the deeper reasons behind physical causes of disease and began working with emotions to improve people's health.

I investigated chakras, the etheric body, and our energetic templates. Our bodies hang on to limiting beliefs from childhood, inherited beliefs, and other traits that become stored in our DNA down through the generations.

Nearly thirty years and four kids later, I now have a greater understanding of the amazing ability of our bodies' ability to heal.

Our body is like a car, and we are in the driver's seat telling it where to go. Just like a car, your body needs regular service and tune-ups. It requires regular maintenance to keep it functioning at its optimal level.

Healing ourselves requires collaboration and teamwork holistically from our mind, body, and soul. After all, team work makes the dream work.

WHY DO YOU THINK IT'S SO IMPORTANT FOR PEOPLE TO BE AWARE OF HOW THE BODY HEALS ITSELF?

You can work with your body to give it what it wants! Your body has the ability to talk to you and let you know what's not working and where it needs you to pay attention.

I have this saying *Listen to your body because it's got something to say.* The more you turn a blind eye to what needs addressing, the louder your body is going to scream at you to wake up and make a change.

Your body is a vessel that physically sends messages to you to wake up and take note. When you're feeling stressed, for example, you might break out in eczema or get butterflies in your tummy. If you're feeling unhappy or depressed, then you may be tired, sluggish, or unmotivated. How you're feeling is linked to what's going on inside your body.

You can't change what you don't know. If you have a conscious awareness of what's going on in your body, then you can do something about it. You can focus your attention and energy to release what is stuck there.

I've taken a lot of courses and read a lot of books about the body's innate ability to heal. I have heard many amazing stories and met lots of incredible people. Some of the healing stories from Dr. Joe Dispenza's work are mind-blowing.

The more you connect with all levels of your body—physical, mental, emotional, spiritual, and dimensional—the greater connection you have to alignment and flow, not just for wellness but for the prevention of future illness. You can have wellness on all of these levels.

You have the ability to heal yourself physically. Just as importantly, you have the ability to heal the way you feel about yourself on the inside. With every healing comes a lesson to be learnt.

Become a private detective of your own body. Start investigating your deeper layers and find that conscious connection with yourself. *Why am I ill in the first place? Where am I out of alignment? What could be a deeper reason for it? What can I do now to improve my quality of life?* Healing requires doing the deeper inner work.

Begin with finding peace within yourself and accept what's going on in your body. One of the biggest facilitators to healing pain is to step away from the stress and into the peace.

You have the ability to enhance wellness or illness by your attitude and intentions. Perception is everything, and you can perceive everything that happens to you to be either positive or negative. Two very different energies.

When you do the INside work, you will soon stop looking outside for the answers, and find them within yourself. When you have a conscious connection to your body, you can unite the three aspects of mind, body, and soul to collaborate.

Your health is your responsibility, and the greater awareness you have of your body, how it can talk to you and heal, and the more you take ownership of it, then you can improve your health and prevent future illness.

WHAT ADVICE DO YOU HAVE FOR CREATING HEALTH AND VITALITY FROM THE INSIDE OUT?

Listen to your body. Get in tune with what it does and doesn't like. Listen to what it's telling you. If you have a niggling suspicion or something doesn't feel right, connect with that feeling and become your own detective. Find that connection inside to what's going on at a deeper level. When you feel out of alignment, have a look at what's causing that and what you need to do to get back to stability and flow. Ask your body questions and listen to what it says.

Commit to taking responsibility for your health and well-being. It's your body, so own it. Do the inner work; make your health a priority, especially around your mind and your mindset, your body, your gut, and your soul. Do the things that bring you joy and make your soul sing.

Your *power* is inside of you, not outside of you.

Attitude is everything. Choose to have a healthy, positive mindset. The choice is yours every single day. Everything can be perceived in a negative or positive way. Maintaining a positive mindset, and staying positive in your thoughts, feelings, and actions, is essential.

Where your thoughts go, your energy flows. What you think, you become.

Be mindful of your words and thoughts because they are energy and, consequently, very powerful. What you think, you create. Focus on what's important to you. Let all that other stuff go.

Think about the thoughts you are putting into your head. What are those thoughts creating in your body? Are they loving, caring, nurturing thoughts or are they self-destructive and negative thoughts?

Your mind chatter is crucial in creating a healthier internal environment. Step up and become your inner coach and push your inner critic to the side. Your autopilot response is to put yourself down and self-sabotage. But if you *stop, pause,* and take time to *respond* rather than *react*, then you have an opportunity to shift your mindset into the light and out of the dark.

Live by my mantra: *Let Go, Step Up, and Be More.*

Let go of hanging around people who don't serve you. Walk away from unhealthy situations. Implement some boundaries. Say no to the draining energies and yes to the uplifting ones. *Let go so you can flow!*

Step up into choices that empower and strengthen you and align with who you truly are and are choosing to be. Relax more. Stress less.

Be more of you—of your authentic self. Speak your truth. Shine your light. Be a beacon of love and light.

Hang around like-minded people—people who have similar beliefs. Workshop life with your friends. Bring your stuff up and out. I like to do that while working out with my girlfriends.

Have an accountability buddy who can support, inspire, and motivate you to stay on track. You can do the same for them.

Listen or read empowering podcasts or books while walking in nature

Live your life with balance because, after all, we are human beings here on earth trying to live a more spiritual and aligned life. I like to try the 80/20 rule: 80% on track and 20% a little wobbly!

Don't hang on to emotions and amplify them by creating drama or stories that become stored in your body. Allow emotions to flow through you. Sometimes you just have to write the day off and remember that tomorrow is a new day, and you can reset. It's amazing to see people change and become so much lighter when they let go and release old, stored emotions.

Be comfortable in your own skin and with the choices you make. Own them. Try to live a more spiritual and aligned life whilst navigating your way through the day-to-day challenges.

Connect holistically with your mind, body, and soul and work as a team collectively. Remember *Team work makes the Dream work!*

Have absolute gratitude for your body and how amazing it is. Every day let your body know how grateful you are for all that it does to support you.

Embrace and immerse yourself with wellness activities, like meditation and walking in nature, bringing it back to basics. What brings you joy and happiness? Do more of that!

Connect with your senses — like oils, sprays, essences, and fresh flowers. Use crystals, listen to music, play frequencies, have a massage, or take an Epsom salt bath.

Make the choice to create positive change in your life and become your own private detective to investigate what's going on inside of you. As my business tagline says, *Empower Yourself Inside and Out!* That will make you Holistically Fit!

About the Author

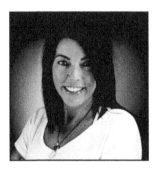

Sally Estlin is a Holistically Fit specialist based in Melbourne, Australia. Her passion is helping people *Let Go, Step Up, and Be More,* to live a more stable, aligned, and purposeful life. She helps people break through barriers to create positive change.

Sally founded Holistically Fit following her love for health, fitness, and general well-being. It started as a personal training business and evolved to focus on deeper personal growth and energy healing. Based on her experience and in-depth learnings, particularly with natural therapies and alternative medicine, her interest is working with the whole individual integrating the mind, body, and soul.

Sally incorporates a myriad of tools and techniques. Her services include personal training, hands-on healing, online coaching, and remote energy work.

Sally has published a 30-day Wellness Mindset Journal, offers intuitive card readings, and is a Wellness Coach and change agent, personal trainer, podcaster, and cohost on an international networking group HNP. She hosted *Your Holistically Fit Life* on the Natural TV channel, RokuTV, and e360TV, and she has launched an Empowered Clothing range.

Sally is guided by her intuition and follows the energy. She has four amazing kids and loves being in nature, exercising, and workshopping life.

Visit her websites holisticallyfit.com.au or empoweredclothing.com.au

Or email: sally@holisticallyfit.com.au

Are you a Worrier or a Warrior? Take the test: holisticallyfit.com.au/warriortest

Order your Wellness Mindset Journal: holisticallyfit. com.au/journal/

Let's have a chat! holisticallyfit.com.au/book-a-call/

Dr. Karen Kan G

WHEN AND HOW DID YOU FIRST DISCOVER THE BODY HAS THE INNATE ABILITY TO HEAL ITSELF?

I have always been fascinated, even as a child, by how a cut heals itself. I didn't understand why it worked and thought that going to school to learn biology, physiology, and biochemistry would explain it. But it didn't. Then I went to medical school, curious as to why some people healed easily and others didn't. Unfortunately, the more I studied, the more indoctrinated I became to thinking that something outside of us was necessary to heal. Now, I've come full circle.

Having witnessed thousands of people learning how to heal themselves by rebalancing their energy, I'm back to my childhood fascination with self-healing. I am grateful that I get to learn, heal, and teach in this amazing playground called life.

Why do you think it's so important for people to be aware of how the body heals itself?

When I began medical school, I was smart, bright-eyed, and caring. I was also extremely naïve. I was completely unaware of the medical-industrial complex that conditions us to believe that the body is a faulty machine and bad genes are the cause of most medical conditions.

Like most of my classmates, I passionately wanted to help people. In school, we focused on diseases and everything that could go wrong with the body instead of focusing on what made people well. In fact, we rarely acknowledged our own self-healing mechanisms. None of our professors really knew how to teach that subject.

Now that I have learned a lot more about how consciousness, energy, and spirituality affect the health of the human body, I'm passionate about sharing this wisdom with others so they do not have to suffer the myriad of diseases that are absolutely preventable and reversible.

If we believe that only something outside of ourselves can heal us, we will be at the mercy of those who stand to gain financially from our ignorance. The war on cancer has produced more cancer. The war on drugs has produced more addiction. The war on fat has produced more obesity and heart disease. When will we wake up and realize that our consciousness, when focused on what we do not desire, will create more of what we do not desire: war, illness, poverty, and more?

It is more important than ever that the wisdom in these pages is shared far and wide. Imagine a world where everyone can tap into and amplify their own natural healing powers. We would stop worrying about other people and take responsibility for ourselves. We would no longer be victims of a medical system whose purpose doesn't seem to be creating health but creating long-term customers.

Let's be clear. I am not anti-medicine or anti-science. Quite the opposite. I am pro-freedom of choice, and I am pro whatever works. Everyone is unique and only the individual can know what is best for him or herself. Conventional medicine has its place. It isn't the enemy.

There are times when conventional medicine shines, especially in emergency life-threatening situations. Combining conventional medicine with the knowledge of how to optimize our own self-healing mechanisms will revolutionize medicine, shifting it from being focused solely on sick care to creating health care. Why spend billions of dollars on a fancy new injectable drug with potential side effects when we can save more lives and increase quality of life by ensuring the availability of nutritious food, clean water, and sanitation for all humans on the planet?

WHAT ADVICE DO YOU HAVE FOR CREATING HEALTH AND VITALITY FROM THE INSIDE OUT?

There is no question that creating health is an inside job. No one needs to fix you, and you don't need to be rescued.

First, realize that who you are is not the body you see reflected in the mirror. You are much more than that. You are a fractal of the Infinite, a spiritual being having a human experience. Even if your body dies, *you* cannot die. Eliminating your fear of death and annihilation is one of ways you can stay level-headed and sovereign throughout all your personal health decisions.

Second, your resonance informs your biology. That means that the quality of your overall energy signature, including the energetic environment that you choose to participate in, tells your DNA and cells what to do. If you are resonating despair and victimhood, different proteins are made from your DNA versus if you are resonating love and peace. This phenomenon is called epigenetics and was first discovered by Dr. Bruce Lipton in the 1960s.

Third, go to Stillness as often as you can throughout your day, even if it is only for a few seconds at a time. This doesn't mean you have to be sitting still with your eyes closed, although many people start learning it that way. It means focusing your mind on being fully present and being fully embodied. Being fully embodied is easiest when you can pay attention to the energy or movement inside your body. I call this technique STOIM, *stillness through observing internal movement*. The mind stills as it focuses awareness on the body. After working with thousands of people, I've come to acknowledge that STOIM helps you access the autohealing state.

The autohealing state is a state of beingness that optimizes the self-healing of organs, glands, cells, and more. The Heartmath Institute calls this state *coherence*, and it can be measured by tracking the electrical signals of the heart and brain simultaneously. There are many ways to reach Stillness. Heartmath teaches one way and I teach another. Both methods are doorways to Stillness and the autohealing state. Choose whatever method(s) work best for you.

The benefits of Stillness not only affect physical healing but multidimensional healing, which includes the mental, emotional, energetic, spiritual, and dimensional aspects of who we are. Stillness also gives us access to our deepest intuitive wisdom. By learning to be fully present and embodied, we can receive Source guidance directly into our awareness. If you ever feel confused or anxious, go to Stillness and allow the answer to drop in. The answer is often gentle, neutral, and fleeting, so be alert and aware.

Our culture is so enamored with the latest flashy app, gadget, or method, that we can easily overlook the simplicity of Stillness as an effective (and inexpensive) path to true health and wellness.

About the Author

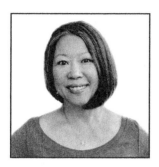

Dr. Karen Kan G is a Doctor of Light Medicine™, a #1 international bestselling author, visionary, and pioneer in healing, consciousness, and spirituality.

Her mission is to empower spiritually conscious people to harness their intuitive, healing, and manifest Superpowers to reach their highest vibration so they can help anchor the new reality of Heaven on Earth.

As the Founder of the Academy of Light Medicine, Dr. Karen teaches students her three-step TOLPAKAN Healing Method (TKH) which involves *aligning* with the Source of Divine Wisdom, *asking* quality questions through Divine Muscle Testing, and *activating* high vibrational healing frequencies. She is like Yoda from *Star Wars*, training you to be a self-healing Jedi Master.

Get into the autohealing state by learning the STOIM technique for free. It can be found at StillnessOnTheFly. com.

Connect with Dr. Karen and other like-minded spiritual evolutionists in the Light Medicine Community. Membership is free: KarenKan.com/LMCfree

Mark Hattas, PhD (h.c.)

WHEN AND HOW DID YOU FIRST DISCOVER THE BODY HAS THE INNATE ABILITY TO HEAL ITSELF?

My mind opened to the possibility that I could heal myself in 2011. I had gone through a manic experience, for the first time, and I was told by doctors that there was absolutely no cure and to plan on being heavily medicated for the rest of my life. It did not ring true to me, but for three years I followed mainstream protocols.

The process that I was told I needed to be on was not helping me get well. I hit a low during my third hospitalization after being diagnosed with bipolar 1 disorder. It was then I decided if I am going to live, I am *actually going to live*. I fired my doctor who had rejected a natural remedy and started seeking alternative solutions. That was when I realized I could get healthy. The alternative solutions led to full restoration of my health.

I have been off all medications since 2015, and I love bringing hope to people who have found themselves in a similar situation. As I got healthy, my *inner GPS system* was activated, and I have since learned that is innate within every human being. My life now is integrated in a whole way, and I trust my *inner GPS system* more and more.

Prior to coming into conscious possession of my inner knowing I thought this type of guidance came from outside of me, and it felt very random. My healing process brought about an integration, almost merging the idea that it is out there with the reality that it was really coming through me. That was amazing and something I love talking about because if we can learn to activate, refine, and trust our inner guidance system, we will be led to optimal outcomes in our physical, mental, emotional, and spiritual health and well-being. I have countless stories of that being a real thing, not just for myself but for many people whom I have seen or guided through the process. It is so fun and enjoyable. It is like the lights go on and life becomes more awe-inspiring.

Why do you think it's so important for people to be aware of how the body heals itself?

With our nonprofit and for-profit corporations, we see many people struggling, and it is common for people to be on protocols that are intended to be helpful but are not. I feel like there is a secret that I did not know for forty years of my life. I am fifty now. Since I experienced the unveiling of this secret, I want everyone to know about it. It does not mean you should not take your medication or should not have a surgery or not do something that is in your highest and best interest. Quite the opposite. It is to be present fully in alignment with the truth of who we are and trust the path that is in your highest and best interest. That will be very different for each person, and countless examples exist.

I was led to the right doctors, programs, technologies, and tools to support healing my gut, getting the proper nutrients to the brain, and unwinding distortions in my mind; and that was just the start. Today, the insights come constantly. I will share just one that was very recent.

A friend of mine had been contacted by someone in Colorado speaking on mental health. Based on the topic, my friend told him, "You have to talk to Mark Hattas. If there is one person to talk to, you have to talk to Mark Hattas."

The guy reached out, we spoke a little bit, and he said "Hey, there is a medical event happening near you in two days, and this amazing doctor will be there," and Mr. Colorado thought I might enjoy listening to him.

I went, and it opened my mind to so much more and was perfectly suited for my interests. I looked at how that came about and wondered, *Why did I go? I do not go listen to doctors' presentations; I am not in the medical field. Why would I go do that?* But my intuition was super sharp, and I just knew I needed to go; it was a game changer. If you can get to a stage where you know you are centered and you are in tune with your highest and best self and allow for the innate guidance to be online and purified, that guidance from love is going to always, one hundred percent of the time, lead you to your best outcomes. Everyone needs to know that is possible and within their grasp.

WHAT ADVICE DO YOU HAVE FOR CREATING HEALTH AND VITALITY FROM THE INSIDE OUT?

If you do not trust your innate guidance system or have access to it or believe you have access to it, learn the skills to activate that guidance and learn the methods to stay in that centered optimal state, that whole state, where you have access to infinite intelligence. Let your desire to be well grow. Give yourself permission to let your desire really be there. It is something that may have been squelched out of you.

One person I spoke with about the possibility of being well said, "Mark, since I was eleven years old, the doctor has told me to take this little white pill and I would be okay." And her belief system prevented her from opening up to anything that contradicted what her doctor told her. Today I would say to her, "Maybe it is time to find a second opinion."

If you let this desire grow, and you learn some skills and start activating your guidance system, you will start tuning into where your inner guidance is leading your life, and it always leads you to health, well-being, and your best most fulfilling life. It is designed that way. It is like gravity. If I drop something, it is going to fall. It is a law of physics. Our human system is designed to support our highest and best interests. Our resistance keeps it from functioning properly. By activating this guidance system, your healing increases, your resistance lowers, and your personal code becomes refined.

Your personal code is an automatic decision designed to serve you when it is aligned. If it is out of alignment, you can retrain it. Your personal code is made up of ten elements of effectiveness and well-being. As your personal code becomes refined, your automatic reactions and patterns fall away so you can consistently show up in your presence, your optimal state. It's incredible to see life change as your personal code changes.

Find a support group of people who are like-minded and going through the activation and restoration process too. As you grow in your experiences, you can support each other. That trust will build within you and within the people in your group. That creates a massive exponential multiplier effect.

When I look at how I spend my time with our coaching services, programs, tools, and training, I realize I am compelled: This is the number one thing for me to do on this planet. I remember when I was far removed from accessing my guidance system. I distrusted it and lost touch with my true self, which led to my mental health issues. As I came back online, so to speak, my mental health issues completely went away. It can happen for you as well. Not everyone will get to the identical level of health and vitality, but you will reach the highest level of health and vitality that is possible for you. May your journey to your best life, including your health, be spectacular!

About the Author

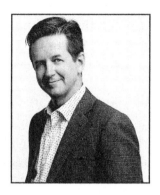

Mark Hattas, PhD (h.c.)

Mark Hattas helps people become the very best they can be. As a certified mental performance coach, he works with executives, entrepreneurs, actors, athletes, and individuals to tune in to the best of who they are and stay there consistently. Mark helps people shed issues and anything else that blocks them from realizing their potential—skills he acquired from navigating his own crisis.

After Mark built and sold a tech company, he navigated a bipolar 1 diagnosis. Doctors told him there was no cure and that medication was his only option. That turned out to be untrue. Today he is healthy and takes no medication. His path to health included physical, mental, emotional, and spiritual healing. The tools

Mark learned he now shares through books, programs, coaching, and speaking.

Mark is a six-time author, including two international bestsellers, co-creator of the Optimal Being program, co-founder of Journey's Dream, a 501(c)3 for mental health, and co-founder of Discover Ancient Wisdom.

Mark was recently conferred an honorary PhD in Entrepreneurship and Business from Trinity University of Ambassadors (TIUA) School of Business, recognizing his achievements in executive and mental performance coaching, entrepreneurship, business, and charitable contributions to mental health.

There are so many resources he wants to share with you, and many of them are free. Go to journeysdream. org/inside to access all of them. May your journey to health be one of glorious returns!

Patra Healey, LMT, CST-T

WHEN AND HOW DID YOU FIRST DISCOVER THE BODY HAS THE INNATE ABILITY TO HEAL ITSELF?

In 2004, I was diagnosed and hospitalized for bipolar with psychotic episodes. Every nightmare I ever imagined came crashing in on me, debilitating every aspect of my being. I heard myself say, "I knew it. My brain is broken, and I have gone crazy." That was the most difficult week of my life. Many antipsychotics, antidepressants, and antianxiety meds were pumped into me. I lost my appetite, couldn't sleep, and had no privacy. Even with a broken brain, I still had enough intelligence to convince the doctors I was well enough to go home. My family was at a loss as to what to do with or for me. I was listless and lost and felt very alone and confused. My emotions were completely out of control, and the medications made me apathetic.

Seven years later, I found a natural neurologist who helped me discover that my body was riddled with candida. That discovery brought on an unraveling that delivered me onto the path I am today.

We found that chronic Lyme disease plagued my body. I was wracked with insurmountable pain, fatigue, and misery. Lyme was affecting my body and my emotions, and it had invaded my brain. I had cognitive difficulties and was emotionally out of control. For the next year, I went back to conventional medicine, which provided absolutely no change. In many ways, my health was worse. Continual antibiotic intake destroyed my gut and caused massive hair loss, cognitive dysfunction, and physical instability. I became bed-bound for three months and was given intravenous antibiotics.

Three nights in a row, I had visions of who I believed to be Jesus, floating over me, sending bright light into my being to heal me. The visions continued sporadically over the next few weeks.

I had been straddling the world of holistic healing and conventional treatment. Shortly after my visions, I decided I needed to find another way. I was insistent the God I know doesn't create mistakes or junk and has given us everything we need in this life. I began a quest to heal myself. I never looked back, and I made continual, incremental steps forward.

Amazing, experienced, and wise people came into my life and taught me new approaches and ways of living. It became clear to me that discovering the ancient paths was the only way to find what I was looking for. I began studying the diets and ways of ancient peoples, discovering that they seemed to have an understanding about the world around them, synchronicity with the cycles of nature, and a perspective on the earth that's been lost in the modern times. I also noticed a steady link between different types of meditation, including meditative movement, and an overall sense of well-being. After changing my diet, adding supplements, implementing multiple healing modalities, homeopathic remedies, and essential oils, I had glimpses that my body was a perfect creation and can grant me all the answers I need. I just need to listen. I have gained a progressive understanding and continue to learn more.

Early on in my craniosacral therapy work, while learning to access the inner physician in my clients and myself, deep truths were revealed and unforeseen healing occurred. Miracles were unfolding before my eyes. A remembering was happening that gave allowance for me to dive further into this unknown world within. I became passionately inspired to discover more.

Several years ago, I was struggling to resolve a health issue. I questioned everyone I knew and sought out naturopaths, therapists, colleagues, and trusted friends. Then one afternoon, it was as if all the wisdom I learned over the years suddenly came together. I realized that I have all the answers I need. In that moment, I fell on my knees and wept. I was overwhelmed with gratitude and encouragement. There was always a very prayerful and spiritual aspect to my life, but that moment led to a deep sense of the need for quiet meditation, daily mindfulness, and a connection with the source of all things. My intuition has continued to develop and guide every step I take to heal my body.

At that point, my physical healing was much improved, but I was still struggling with depression, anxiety, and a lack of contentment. Through my craniosacral training, I was very familiar with SomatoEmotional Release (SER), developed from Carl Jung's research. I began applying it to myself in meditation, playing the roles of therapist and client. It was interesting to learn that I am more than just the thoughts that run through my mind or the emotions that flood my body in response to events. There are multiple parts of me that live in my body along with a wise observer who can see it all.

I sat back during these meditative times and observed everything that came into my awareness. Deep emotional pain washed through my body, wave after wave, until I became calm again. I accessed painful areas and discovered intense traumas that lived within me. Eventually, I was able to discover a place of deep inner stillness and knowing. This was the most powerful place I've discovered, internally or externally. It's in the stillness that the quiet, small voice speaks clearly to me, giving me guidance, direction, and wisdom.

Sometimes, I find very clear direction. Other times, the guidance leads me to take specific steps throughout the day or brings people into my life to teach me, love me, support me, and accept me. The discoveries have been small and incremental, giant leaps, or steadily unfolding as I move forward in my journey of self-discovery. My inner wisdom leads the way as I continue to move more in flow with the universe.

The stillness has begun to permeate my daily life, giving me a solid place to return to during chaotic times and a steady diving platform as I engage with limitless possibilities.

Stillness has become my touchstone from where every decision, step, and dream unfold. I return to stillness again and again, discovering deeper places of amazing truths. Every time I move into stillness, which can be for a minute or two throughout the day, during sessions with my clients, or in a more traditional mediation, I can feel myself connecting more clearly with the Divine that resides inside of me and connects me to all others. There is absolute truth to Psalm 46:10, "Be still and know that I am God."

I continue my healing work with my acupuncturist, other craniosacral practitioners, naturopaths, and energy healers. They are all amazing supports and help me reset so I can continue to move forward. I often remind my clients when they get frustrated about being stuck or can't get through something, that we can't do it all on our own. We need each other and sometimes we need a professional to help.

In this rat race culture, stillness and looking inward seem so counter intuitive. But the ancients knew differently. Many religions and cultures discuss meditation, prayer, stillness, and quiet. Connecting with yourself and your Higher Power, if you believe in one, is the foundation of leading a full life. It is the wellspring that feeds your soul.

WHY DO YOU THINK IT'S SO IMPORTANT FOR PEOPLE TO BE AWARE OF HOW THE BODY HEALS ITSELF?

To discover your own innate ability to heal is probably the most powerful understanding you can have in this life. By knowing and accessing this wisdom, you are able to bring healing, wisdom, guidance, and love into a world full of the broken hearted and hurting. Not only can you heal yourself, but you can heal the world. We need each other for connection and nurturing, and you can trust that the wisdom that lies in your teacher, leader, pastor, counselor, or therapist also lies within you. Accessing your inner wisdom is beneficial for your own healing journey, and it is an expansive experience for you and those around you. It is like throwing a pebble into a pond; the ripple effect is profound and unending.

Taking back your power is going to positively impact your health, relationships, career, personal time, lifestyle, and the way you function in your community. When you value a relationship, you spend time with that person, getting to know them, what they like, and who they are. The relationship you have with yourself is just as important and the most valuable relationship you can invest in. Spending time with yourself, listening and exploring who you are, is the most important thing you can do for those you love. Loving and caring for yourself allows you to bring the best version of you to any relationship.

WHAT ADVICE DO YOU HAVE FOR CREATING HEALTH AND VITALITY FROM THE INSIDE OUT?

Allow yourself to experiment with trial and error. Learn and keep moving forward. There is no such thing as failure in this situation. Discover how you connect with yourself. Some people need to engage in quiet activities such as puzzles, gardening, walking, sewing, cooking, or some other hobby. You have the answers you need. There is no right or wrong way, just your way.

I enjoy doing puzzles, cooking, nanograms, and staring at the pond outside my window. I do some QiGong and silent mediation too. I step into stillness throughout the day, just to check in and see how I'm doing. It's like sending a love note to my significant other. "How are you? Doing okay? I love you."

Some ways to connect with yourself:

- Get quiet. Be with yourself, your body, your pain.

- Sit in your favorite chair, outside or in nature with your phone turned off.

- Go for a walk.

- Listen and observe. You are not your thoughts or your emotions. Listen to your body.

- The pain, screaming anxiety, or deafening depression need your attention. Put your awareness or mind's eye into these places and observe. Acknowledge them and allow them to exist. Observe everything. The thoughts. The feelings. The pain.

- If emotions come up, feel them through to the end. Do not suppress them.

- Be gracious and gentle with yourself. No judgment. No agenda. Just be.

- Find a professional skilled in somatic emotional therapy to support you on your journey.

About the Author

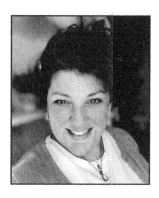

Self-healing is something Patra is very familiar with. After receiving a diagnosis of bipolar with psychotic episodes in 2004 and Lyme disease in 2010, she found herself on a pursuit of health that led her to craniosacral therapy (CST). Through the use of Young Living therapeutic essential oils, the Weston A. Price diet, supplements, CST, and other healing modalities, she has fully recovered from bipolar and Lyme and is living a passion-filled life. On this journey, she discovered inner healing and her passion to support others who are seeking the same.

Being fully recovered from these diagnoses, she continues to learn, heal, and grow. Licensed in the state of Maryland, Patra is a Techniques Certified Craniosacral Therapist with a focus on SomatoEmotional Release work and brings all her experience to her online healing sessions with clients. It is her deepest desire to support others in self-discovery and facilitate their journey of self-healing.

Patra enjoys time with her rescued Chihuahua mix Oliver, expanding with her Dream Weaving Loom, cooking nourishing food, solving puzzles of all sorts, and engaging in deep conversation with friends. Patra has carved out a quiet, peaceful, connected lifestyle that moves at the pace she desires.

If you are interested in working with Patra or learning more, please visit patrahealey.com or send an email to patracst@gmail.com.

For more of Patra's internal healing journey, click the blog tab on her website patrahealey.com.

Cathy Hohmeyer

WHEN AND HOW DID YOU FIRST DISCOVER THE BODY HAS THE INNATE ABILITY TO HEAL ITSELF?

I grew up in a rural environment where health services were limited, and the tradition of health care was based on more natural ingredients and processes. I saw from an early age that the body is able to heal itself. Our town was literally built for tuberculosis patients who came for their cure based on the few medical remedies available at the time. Those Adirondack Mountains in northern New York state came to be known as the Healing Woods.

While studying energetics, I investigated traditional methods of self-healing and was astounded by the wealth of knowledge and practices that were used in many civilizations. Not all of these practices have been abandoned. The ancient Egyptians used sound healing and Tibetan Buddhists continue to do so today. Sound healing has found its way to the west and is used in many healing practices. Quantum physicists define sound healing as energetic medicine.

Little did I know that I would have to go through this process myself. I discovered I was ill and compromised, unusual for me.

In a matter of a week, I resolved to self-heal or bust. First, I needed to get through the fear instilled by a lifetime in the system.

By knowing the software of my body blueprint, I knew steps to calm the uneven heartbeats and to reset my body to healing mode. Next, I analyzed my voice print. Your body might know what it needs to do but without proper nourishment it cannot accomplish it. Nourishment is not about following a diet or nutritional rules. It is about getting what you need when you need it. And that means multidimensionally.

WHY DO YOU THINK IT'S SO IMPORTANT FOR PEOPLE TO BE AWARE OF HOW THE BODY HEALS ITSELF?

The human body is an amazing creation that possesses a wellness toolbox containing the power of mind, spirit, and body. When balance is challenged, each person's toolbox along with nature can re-create wellness within. This renders humans capable of creating their own MD, or Multi-Dimensional healing.

Using my background as an occupational therapist (OTR) my toolbox contains innovative ways to arrive at a solution. For example, a client loved to do macramé before she injured her arm, so the OTR set up an exercise to strengthen the arm, using a macrame task. A therapist will use each client's skills and abilities to create the best amount of independence for that person.

It is possible to strengthen the mind and spirit to assist in the rehabilitation process. This includes incorporating healthy foods into the diet and upping your energetic spirit.

Many physical problems are a result of the interconnectedness of mind and spirit. Physical ailments can often be an outgrowth of poor diet, a response to stress like divorce or other mental/emotional stressors, or a consequence of outside energies. It is key to know our biological laws.

Accidents, malnutrition, and poisoning assuredly need immediate measures. But much of what we call dis-ease are actually healing reactions on an ancient reactive level—an integrated safety mechanism involving the psyche, the brain, and the connected organ.

WHAT ADVICE DO YOU HAVE FOR CREATING HEALTH AND VITALITY FROM THE INSIDE OUT?

When you work with this amazing biological mechanism, it will sustain you on a daily basis by growing, repairing cells, losing cells or even reducing the function of a system. These are temporary *software programs* your body uses to keep you safe when unexpected events occur. Recognizing these programs is one of the keys to your best form of self-knowing.

Everything is energy and energy is frequency. You can learn to decipher frequencies and to multidimensionally nourish yourself to improve your life force. You can be your own energy and your own life force creator.

While we are taught in school about basic biology and immune systems, there is often not an emphasis on how the body, mind, and spirit comprise a self-healing machine. Let's think for the moment about the self-healing our body does each moment of every day. Our intestines process nutriment and remove the detritus. Our brain analyzes wounds and directs the manufacture of appropriate *cell doctors* to heal them. Glands balance endorphins based on mental stress and direct how to process the meal you just ate.

Why, then, would the body — and its wellness partners spirit and mind — not be able to fix itself on other fronts? While self-healing may not always be the answer to all wellness questions, an approach that abandons your ability to self-heal is self-sabotage.

We have been taught to call on others or on physical tools to fix what might be perceived as broken within us. Looking deeper, you find the ability inside ... the ability to use the amazing *inner software* that you were born with but may not have recognized until now. Continually relying on other people or tools only makes you more dependent. What if that other person isn't there? What if your equipment is missing or broken? Augment yourself with tools and slowly integrate the knowing that you can go it alone.

If you know what you need to nourish your body, your body *knows* what to do with it. I have learned to nourish myself and others by delving into the body blueprint and seeing the frequencies within. Humans are an amazing array of mathematical frequencies that produce a unique hue-man.

Just as the universe has universal laws to maintain its ultimate structure through thick and thin, your body has biological laws. Keeping those in mind, you can know the frequencies that you need in a day. As the late genius Lloyd Mear instructed, some frequencies are in tune, some out of tune, and some are missing.

I work with intuition and voice print capabilities that render vast amounts of vibrational information. Just imagine, when you get up in the morning you *know* what you need to keep your body balanced! You can know what supplements you need, what muscle is imbalanced, and even what color of food is beneficial for you. What a day you could have! What a week! What a life!

Sound is considered a healing modality. But do you know the depths of its knowledge for you? You can know your individuality by looking at how our frequencies are working together in your body. Sound is an amazing tool to have in your box.

There are people described as *breatharians* who eat and drink very little but still remain healthy. While I love food, I have experienced a phase of this in part via bioacoustic frequency analysis and programming. At one point, I couldn't walk the stairs without placing a frequency of oxygen in my field via programming it to a *tone box* and listening to a headset. My compromised lungs filled with air and my somersaulting heart calmed down as the tones filled me. I could feel my lungs fill with air just like taking a deep breath.

Nourish your third body with nutrient-dense foods proven to have made our ancestors healthy beyond most of our generation. These foods are full of enzymes, vitamins, and nutrients, made in a very simple, easy, and cost-effective process.

Re-establish the energetic relationship of food. Peoples' blueprints have been compromised, and food also. Let's get our foods back to the divine blueprint and learn to bring in as much Life Force as possible. And no, you do not need to be live food or totally plant based.

Reliance on technology reduces your intuition. Although you can use the amazing technology as a learning tool and learn from it while developing your own inner skills. It's easy to rely on technology alone to tell you what is wrong or possibly how to fix it. But you need to remember to always rely on improving your own amazing "super powers" and to keep learning more about and how to use your quantum bio-software within.

For a free voice analysis to see how you can begin to "Know Yourself Through Frequency" or to learn some of the secrets of your own Body Software programs, contact Cathy at info@lakeclearlodge.com or see the property for yourself at lakeclearlodge.com and watch a spectacular sunset over the portal, lake, and mountains at lakeclearlodge.com/webcam. Cathy may be in the kitchen creating energized foods, online with a client, or teaching classes at the retreat center, and she would love to hear from you.

About the Author

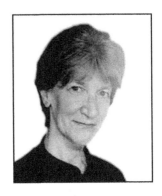

Cathy grew up running in the woods and swimming in the lakes of the Adirondack Mountains. After earning her degree in Occupational Therapy, she began working in Washington DC. After a few years, nature called, and she returned to her small town and the dream of having a wellness-based resort became clear. Throughout the last thirty-five years, it has been her learning lab to create her program called Nutritional Energetics.

Cathy is a wife, proud mom of three, and owner/ operator of the Lake Clear Lodge, originally built by her great aunt and uncle in 1886. Her family has worked it together, creating a unique space with unique offerings within a whole lot of nature on twenty-five acres and private beachfront, where you can watch a sunset over Saint Regis Mountain.

Cheri Lowman

WHEN AND HOW DID YOU FIRST DISCOVER THE BODY HAS THE INNATE ABILITY TO HEAL ITSELF?

Our bodies are always working toward healing; they just need a little help.

I distinctly recall being in my undergrad anatomy and physiology class, studying the formation of a scab, which results from cutting or scraping our skin. The body immediately begins the formation of a clot on the surface of the skin. It's a very complex process. Simply put, particles called fibrins are sent to the site and pile on each other to form a scab, which stops your body from losing blood and allows the repair process to continue. This was my first discovered profound scientific example of the body's innate power to heal! Healing, like this, is happening on a constant basis all throughout our bodies in a less-visible way.

WHY DO YOU THINK IT'S SO IMPORTANT FOR PEOPLE TO BE AWARE OF HOW THE BODY HEALS ITSELF?

We are all born with a pure innate ability to heal. If we care for our body and provide the support it needs to stay healthy, this process will continue, allowing us to live long, healthy lives.

WHAT ADVICE DO YOU HAVE FOR CREATING HEALTH AND VITALITY FROM THE INSIDE OUT?

Think of yourself as your body's assistant. With just a bit of help, your body can maintain good health. This by itself is important, but it is increasingly important to be able to fight off, or recover from, any illness or injury that might occur.

A few ways you can help your body heal:

Move

Just move. You don't have to exercise strenuously, although that has its benefits. It is important that you are exercising, in some way, on a regular basis. Our bodies are amazingly adaptable! If you are not getting exercise, your body gets the message that you don't need strong muscles and bones. This message is received, and the bones and muscles become weaker. Osteoclasts become abundant and break down bone, resulting in weak and brittle bones, and muscle becomes sarcopenic or wastes.

When you exercise, your body responds by forming new muscle protein strands called microfibers. As you continue to exercise, these microfibers will increase in number and thickness (hypertrophy), resulting in a stronger and larger muscle. Simultaneously, osteoblasts will become more plentiful to build bone, and your bones will become more dense and stronger. This is another example of our body's own instinctive capacity to heal.

Moving after a meal is also important. If you sit after eating, your body will get the message that it needs to store fat. This is why it's necessary to tell your body what to do with your food. Even going for a short walk after eating will let your body know that it's going to be using that food for fuel, not fat.

Eat real food

If you cannot identify it, don't eat it. If it comes in a can or box, it most likely is highly processed and far from being real food. In addition, it probably has preservatives and other added chemicals that can damage your health. Read the label and avoid consumption if there is any ingredient that is not real food. Naturally grown, real foods contain many nutrients and medicinal properties that help your body maintain good health and vitality. These nutrients work on a cellular level to initiate a multitude of chemical and physiological reactions that are important for maintaining general bodily functions.

Make every meal an opportunity for medicine

Every time you eat, whether it is a meal or a snack, is an opportunity to provide nutrients that contribute to your good health. Consider this every single time you consume anything. If you drink a cup of tea, try adding some beneficial herbs or spices. Perhaps add some cinnamon to support blood sugar, reduce inflammation, and help protect against heart disease. Add some clove to improve digestion and help with detoxification. Or add both to spice up your love life! Make your cup of tea or coffee a cup of medicine. You can do the same with salads or most anything when you are making a meal. Remember, if it is not contributing to your health, it is most likely contributing to your demise. We are not sitting still, but always moving either toward or away from good health.

Eating good food takes planning. If you take the time and energy to gather real foods and prepare them correctly, you will have taken a large step toward your longevity.

Avoid these foods

High-fructose corn syrup (HFCS) damages the production of leptin. This is the hormone that is released to provide your body the feeling of satiation or fullness. In other words, leptin tells your body it is full and that you should stop eating. HFCS is also a leading contributor to obesity, inflammation, diabetes, high triglycerides, and non-alcoholic fatty liver disease. It is hidden in many unexpected foods, such as ketchup and barbeque sauce — another good reason to check your labels.

Excessive linoleic acid (LA) consumption is associated with inflammation, obesity, heart disease, and mitochondrial damage. Mitochondria are the powerhouses in our cells that produce energy — adenosine triphosphate (ATP). They are so critical to our health that we would not be alive without them. LA is found in seed oils. There is a particularly high content in safflower, grape, sunflower, corn, cottonseed, soybean, rice bran, peanut, and canola oils. Olive and avocado oils, in their pure form, contain about ten percent LA, making those both better choices. However, it is difficult to find pure oils. Most oils touted as pure olive or avocado oil contain some amount of other less expensive oils. Tallow, butter, or coconut oil contain one to two percent LA and all have additional nutritional benefits. Linoleic acid should be less than two percent of your daily caloric intake.

Use natural remedies

When needed, look for natural remedies that can support your body's innate healing process. As with food, avoid chemical additives or synthetic drugs that may damage your body's instinctive drive to heal. There are many natural and effective resources to assist with ailments that should be considered before succumbing to pharmaceutical options.

Investigate homeopathy

Homeopathy is based on the doctrine like cures like. It is the art of connecting the symptoms, personality, and behaviors of a remedy to that of an individual. Homeopathy is non-invasive and has been found to be helpful for a vast variety of conditions.

Consider constitutional hydrotherapy

An ancient modality that uses applications of wet hot and cold towels to push and pull blood to and from every organ and every cell in the body, this results in increased blood circulation, metabolism, and lymphatic flow, and it stimulates the immune system to speed up the healing process.

Constitutional hydrotherapy is beneficial for anxiety, stress, depression, addiction recovery, weight loss, digestive issues, fatigue, reproductive issues, and many other health issues.

Get the proper amount of sleep

Getting sufficient sleep is one of the most important things we can do for our health. While you are sleeping, a watery liquid called cerebrospinal fluid (CSF) washes through your brain in pulsing waves, cleansing the brain of toxins and other unwanted particles. Many important processes take place while we are sleeping. To ensure your best night's sleep, keep your room dark and remove anything that emits electromagnetic frequencies (EMFs).

Be still

Pencil in a date with yourself each morning. Lie in bed a few moments before you get up. Meditate or just sit with yourself.

Be present. It is in the morning, after a good night's rest, that our bodies are at ease. This is a good time for quiet reflection and connection with spirit. Sit for at least fifteen minutes each morning with no distractions and no phone or other electronics. Allow your true essence to expand and bask in the feeling of who you are. Are you living in alignment with your spirit, your beliefs? Feel into that and make certain you are coordinated with your true self. Give yourself the time and space for reflection. You will find your day evolves with a better sense of direction and flow.

Be grateful

Your morning date is a good time to reflect on what you are grateful for.

Enjoy the little things. For one day you may look back and realize they were the big things.

~Robert Brault

Can you look back at a time *just before* a major tragic event occurred that drastically changed your life? It might have been a death, a loss, an accident, or another experience. Do you recall at that time in your life feeling like life would be better if this or that had happened? What if you made that time now? Look around you at everything you could lose. What if just one of those things was gone tomorrow? Now feel how grateful you are. Embrace anything that is important to you and allow the gratitude to permeate your soul. Be grateful because these are the good ole days.

Gratitude has been scientifically proven to create a stronger immune system, improve blood flow, result in fewer aches and pains, and increase mood and self-satisfaction.

Believe

Believe in yourself.

Henry Ford once said, "Whether you think you can, or think you can't, you're right." We are born into this world and make our way through life influenced by our parents and what they learned from their parents. We are programmed to live following rules that were created by our oldest ancestors who were simply trying to exist. They were foraging for food, fighting off animals, and searching for shelter to rest and recover.

Our whole existence has been based on survival. No one told us that we are beings with unlimited power, and that we are only bound by what we believe. No one told us it's up to us to unleash that power and live to our full potential. Have you heard the story of the mom who pulled the car off her baby? She was able to do that because she stepped beyond the survival belief system. Her love overpowered what she had been taught, and she was able to grasp her true strength. That power is always there, and you have access to that power. You must get past the limits that have been so staunchly instilled in you. Believe that you can, and you will.

If you can come to understand the profound healing naturally taking place in your body and simply help that process along, you will not have to wait for the diagnosis to be your healthiest self!

About the Author

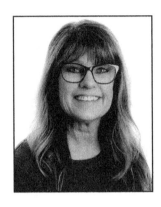

Cheri has studied health-related subjects since she was a small child. She married young, and after raising her family she returned to school, graduating summa cum laude from the University of the Southwest with a bachelor's degree in biology and an emphasis in pre-med. She then attended medical school at Bastyr University where she studied to be a Naturopathic Doctor. While in school, Cheri was the vice president for the San Diego branch of Naturopathic Doctors Without Borders. She received her certification in Homeopathy from the New England School of Homeopathy under Doctors Amy and Paul Herscu. She has studied Energy Healing under Dr. Bradley Nelson and the world-renowned Cyndi Dale.

Cheri and her husband Joel own and direct Healing Springs, in Colorado Springs, Colorado. There she offers Homeopathy, Constitutional Hydrotherapy, and Energy Healing. She is currently working on her first book, titled: *Don't Wait for the Diagnosis*. Cheri has a deep-rooted desire to educate and help people understand they have control over their health, and that small daily habits can dramatically improve their health. It is her goal to help you Be Your Healthiest Self!

For more information on her services, or to book an appointment, please visit hshydro.com or call 719-433-0775.

Remote sessions are available. If you're in Colorado, please stop by!

Don't wait for the diagnosis to be your healthiest self!

Lynne McTaggart

WHEN AND HOW DID YOU FIRST DISCOVER THE BODY HAS THE INNATE ABILITY TO HEAL ITSELF?

In 2007, I started experimenting with the power of group intention. I had written several books about the power of intention and the idea that we're all part of a quantum energy field. I wanted to know how far we could take that power. If thoughts are things that affect other things, what does that mean? Can we cure cancer with our thoughts?

I started experimenting with small groups of eight or so people—something I now call The Power of Eight®. And to my astonishment, I found that when people held an intention for someone else in the group or even outside the group, just for ten minutes, we were healing all manner of things, including cancer and arthritis. Somebody with cataracts was able to see 80 percent better. Two people got out of their wheelchairs. I've done this now with thousands of groups, and I've seen extraordinary healings. For me, it has been demonstrated, without a doubt, that our body has the ability to heal itself with the help of group intention.

WHY DO YOU THINK IT'S SO IMPORTANT FOR PEOPLE TO BE AWARE OF HOW THE BODY HEALS ITSELF?

Modern medicine is failing in anything other than emergency medicine. If I get run over by a truck tomorrow, I want the best of high-tech medicine to put me back together again. But in almost every other regard, like chronic illnesses of any sort, medicine can't heal. It can only maintain the body through drugs that have other side effects.

The body is an extraordinarily complex thing. Even the most sophisticated of artificial intelligence will never approximate the sophistication of the human body with its ability to self-regulate and self-heal. Because our medical tools are so primitive, it's a bit like a caveman being asked to fix a computer. It is important for us to understand how the body heals itself.

WHAT ADVICE DO YOU HAVE FOR CREATING HEALTH AND VITALITY FROM THE INSIDE OUT?

For anything other than emergency medicine, where conventional medicine shines, it's important to understand and be well-versed in the many alternative treatments and integrative treatments that treat the body as a whole person.

It is also important to understand your own power, the power of intention, the power of positive thinking, and the power of intuition. All of these are important for many people in my community when healing the past. The past is sitting in them like an unwanted guest and creating illness. All of these things—understanding the relationship between mind and body, and that we have five pillars of healing, which are diet, supplements, exercise, and also mind and community—all of these things, even community, have a strong ability to heal. To really be well, you must understand the body as a complex, interconnected thing.

About the Author

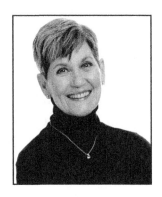

Lynne McTaggart is one of the central authorities on new science and consciousness. She is the award-winning author of seven books, printed in more than thirty languages, including the internationally bestselling *The Intention Experiment, The Field, The Bond and The Power of Eight.*

Lynne is also architect of the Intention Experiments, a web-based global laboratory, and she was prominently featured in the plotline of Dan Brown's blockbuster *The Lost Symbol.*

A highly sought-after public speaker, who has spoken on nearly every continent, Lynne has appeared in many documentaries, including *What the Bleep!?: Down the Rabbit Hole, I Am, The Abundance Factor, The Healing Field, and The 1 Field.*

As co-owner and editorial director of *What Doctors Don't Tell You* (wddty.com), she publishes one of the world's most respected health magazines, now published in fifteen languages. *What Doctors Don't Tell You* has been awarded Best and Most Popular Website of the Year for Health and Well-being and Ethical Business of the Year.

She is consistently listed as one of the world's one hundred most spiritually influential people, and has received multiple awards, including a special award, Champion of Change, from the Unity Church.

Lynne and her husband, WDDTY and Get-Well co-founder Bryan Hubbard, author of the ground-breaking book *The Untrue Story of You*, live in London. They have two adult daughters.

Find out more here:

lynnemctaggart.com

wddty.com

Sylvie Olivier

WHEN AND HOW DID YOU FIRST DISCOVER THE BODY HAS THE INNATE ABILITY TO HEAL ITSELF?

Twenty-five years ago, my daughter was hovering between life and death. It was the second time the doctors had predicted she only had six to seven hours to live. I wanted so much to find a cure for her, and I was at my wit's end, not knowing what to do. I felt desperate. As I cradled her in my arms that night, I whispered gently in her ear, "You know what, Sweetie? If it is too hard for you to continue, I will let you go."

The next morning, she awoke with sparks in her eyes and a liveliness that I had not seen for so long. It took many months for her to make a full recovery, and then the doctor said it was a miracle. When I stopped holding on to her and let her choose from her heart, she came back fully into life.

WHY DO YOU THINK IT'S SO IMPORTANT FOR PEOPLE TO BE AWARE OF HOW THE BODY HEALS ITSELF?

Stop feeling so desperate. Stop seeing yourself as a victim. Stop giving your power to outside sources.

When I realigned myself with my heart, I assisted my daughter to do the same even though she was only five years old at the time. We need to remember who we are and the miracle that we are as human beings. When we allow our heart to take command, everything all around us falls into place. Now when I look at people who are struggling with their health, I have so much compassion for them. People lose their joy of living for many reasons. When I see joy return to their eyes, my heart sings. Realigning with your heart brings a whole lot of opportunities to connect to joy again.

WHAT ADVICE DO YOU HAVE FOR CREATING HEALTH AND VITALITY FROM THE INSIDE OUT?

I love this question because it connects me to my own joy. During the whole process of my daughter's seven-year illness, I studied a lot. I connected with the twelve vibrations of what I received as the Plenitude Effect. These are nine qualities of the heart comprised in three different spheres when your own vibrational signal shifts. It raises and assists you to live with more vitality.

We can talk about love, joy, peace, appreciation, and the courage to listen to the heart. The lightness, compassion, wonder, and care you feel gives you a message — a unique message to your cells that are fed by these vibrations — and vitality returns to you, creating health.

I invite you to open up to receive a side-by-side assistance instead of putting your health in the hands of someone else. Be guided by someone who will assist you to open your heart and naturally connect back to its vibrations. I also invite you to learn about your vibrational signal and how it emits and receives according to your thoughts, your feelings, and your habits. It shifts everything in your posture and the innate ability in your body to restore, rejuvenate, and heal. Invite plenitude in every area of your life and play every single day. I call it the Plenitude Effect with all twelve vibrations, and nothing is missing in Plenitude. There is no lack of health or lack of anything. When you really connect to plenitude, you feel it inside and are co-creating fulfillment in every area of your life.

About the Author

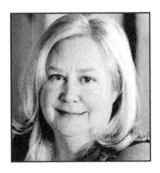

Bioenergetics expert and HeartMath Certified Mentor and Trainer, Sylvie Olivier assists business leaders, professionals, and individuals in experiencing the journey from the head to the heart through private mentoring, programs, and retreats, both online and at live events around the world.

The seriousness of Sylvie's daughter's illness, which lasted seven years, combined with Sylvie's research to find a cure for her daughter, assisted her in facing the obvious. There comes a point when science and conscience meet.

Consequently, through her research, Sylvie discovered that harmonizing the heart and the brain is at the source of this state of Plenitude and optimal health that's naturally available to all human beings.

When we only experience life through our mind, disconnected from the heart, Plenitude is not accessible, therefore creating confusion and disharmony in all spheres of our lives.

Through her research and her journey, Sylvie discovered that human beings naturally possess within them twelve vibrations (nine Heart's Qualities and three Spheres) that are always accessible through the heart: Love, Joy, Peace, Harmony, Appreciation, Courage, Lightness, Vitality, Compassion, Wonder, Care, and Prosperity. These vibrations are at the source of a natural and constant feeling of Plenitude.

Experience the Nine Qualities of the Heart and receive more Harmony, Vitality, and Prosperity with the Plenitude Effect eBook.

This eBook will assist you in connecting and integrating Plenitude into your daily life. Access it by creating a FREE membership here:

goldenheartwisdom.com/en/boutique/free-membership/

Send us an email with "the INside effects" in the subject line and receive free admission to one of our many webinars where you'll be guided to connect to the deepest part of your heart so you can tune in to your purest frequency of health.

Shannon Procise

WHEN AND HOW DID YOU FIRST DISCOVER THE BODY HAS THE INNATE ABILITY TO HEAL ITSELF?

My doctor prescribed a firewalk on a prescription pad. I thought it was very bizarre, but she was adamant I did not have to walk barefoot over the coals; I could just watch. She insisted the experience would be profound and healing for me.

I had given birth to my son Alexander only one week before the event. After watching the first person walk across the coals, something from within told me that I had to walk, too.

The moment I stepped onto the glowing embers, a rush of emotions flooded through me — excitement, trepidation, and a deep sense of connection to something greater than myself. With each step, I could feel the energy of the fire beneath me, a powerful force that seemed to interact with my own energy.

The walk itself was surprisingly swift, lasting only a matter of seconds. The length of the path, six feet, might seem short in the grand scheme of things; but at that moment, it felt like a significant journey. Each step brought me closer to a realization—an understanding that the mind possesses an extraordinary influence over the body's response to the world. It was a profound lesson in the power of belief, resilience, and the innate healing potential that resides within us.

After the firewalk, a newfound passion for the magic of mind over matter was ignited within me. The experience served as a catalyst, awakening a deep curiosity and appreciation for the body's ability to heal itself. It made me realize there are uncharted depths within us, waiting to be explored and tapped into for our well-being and transformation.

Firewalking has been credited with healing cancer and many types of trauma within the body. Learning this inspired me to become a firewalk promoter and host firewalk workshops where I have witnessed many miracles. My favorite is the time I got fire kisses, as they are called—little burns on my feet. A friend, another firewalking instructor, began dancing next to me and said, "Come on. Let's walk together."

I answered her, "Are you crazy?" I was trying to keep my composure because I was the host, but I relented. We walked to the other end, and then the burns were gone. I ended up walking three more times during that event. I became passionate about the magic of that experience of witnessing mind over matter. It gave all of us there that night the courage and power to see how magnificent we are.

Over the years of doing firewalks and helping hundreds of people walk, I have seen profound healing on the physical level, spiritual level, and mental level. I've also seen firewalking kids raise their grades from Fs to As and Bs.

WHY DO YOU THINK IT'S SO IMPORTANT FOR PEOPLE TO BE AWARE OF HOW THE BODY HEALS ITSELF?

The body is a messenger on so many levels. I had multiple surgeries before the age of twenty-one because I had listened to other people. Understanding our body's ability to heal itself takes us from being powerless, losing hope, and being fearful to really understanding and knowing that we have the ability to overcome and create anything, including profound healing. Our body, even beyond our wildest dreams, can do incredible things. It is important to use the body in a positive way and be aware of who we impact. Knowing what the body does and the power it has allows us to be the best we can be, have all the energy that we want, and tap into our intuition.

When we are healthy, whole, and connected with our body, we have an inner guide, an inner voice helping us navigate on a daily basis those challenges, obstacles, and choices that arise when our body is unhealthy or has dis-ease. With health comes power, gifts, and a way to positively affect all of those around us—our family, our business, our friends, and all that we do.

When I am in touch with my body even when it is in discomfort, I am able to tune in to what I need to do. I may need to slow down. I may need to pause. I may be doing something that is not ideal for my journey, my mission, or my path.

Your journey, your mission is yours. Tune into the gifts of your body. I have worked with people who think we are here to dominate the body, and the body has to do what we tell it to do. But really, we are here to become one with our body, understand our body, and listen to our body because every single body is unique. What may be healthy for my body and what my body needs may be the exact opposite of what you may need. And that can change over time as we age or as we grow and have more experiences. This awareness and knowing allows us to tune into our body as a temple for wellness.

WHAT ADVICE DO YOU HAVE FOR CREATING HEALTH AND VITALITY FROM THE INSIDE OUT?

I could write a whole book on this. I use what I call the body pendulum. Some people use a physical pendulum. Other people hear that voice. But the advice I give is to get in touch and strengthen those muscles so you can ask specific questions of yourself. There are so many people trying to tell you to take this vitamin, take this pill, do this process. The fact is your body has an innate wisdom; you have an internal director you continue to block, and you continue to think something may be good for you when it may not be.

For example, I will use the pendulum before I purchase a supplement and ask, "Is this for my highest good right now to take this?" Or I will ask, "Is it for my highest good now to consume this?" Or "Is it for my highest good now to choose this?"

Your body will guide you uniquely and lead you to what is for your highest good, to be able to take actions with certainty when you are given advice. Find a mentor or coach if you are dealing with a health challenge. Find somebody who has been successful overcoming that obstacle. Invest in yourself. Get out of the insurance system and get into the system with people who have experience with wellness and have overcome challenges, so they are at your side and can advocate with you and believe in what you may be learning to believe in yourself, or so they can help you believe in it. Align with someone who will hold that space with you.

About the Author

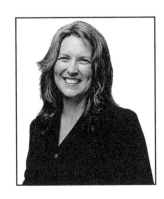

Shannon Procise is the go-to guide for visionaries seeking to create community and cultivate raving fans. Shannon has spent more than two decades building an international business community by helping small businesses grow to their full potential through knowledge-sharing, marketing, and cooperative strategies. A master at creating strategic alliances and developing sustainable partnerships, Shannon almost effortlessly resolves complex issues while motivating teams to peak performance. What's more, she readily shows others how to do the same.

Shannon has appeared on television and radio and in the press. She's co-author of the Amazon #1 bestseller *Law of Business Attraction – The Secret of Cooperative Success* with T. Harv Eker of *The Millionaire Mind*. Shannon is the founder of the Business Acceleration Network, a Trailblazing Community for Conscious Business owners who are here to make an impact. She guides businesses to build successful enterprises while having fun and making lots of money. She brings together social entrepreneurs, visionaries, and new thought leaders who want to collaborate, create a better world, and focus on prosperity so they can pay it forward to make a positive impact.

Join Shannon at www.BodyPendulum.com or MeetShannon.com to explore the innate power of your body to heal itself and learn how the mind-body connection can promote greater wellness. Let's work together to build communities committed to creating positive change in the world through the power of collaboration.

Keith Leon S.

WHEN AND HOW DID YOU FIRST DISCOVER THE BODY HAS THE INNATE ABILITY TO HEAL ITSELF?

When I was a child, my aunt received a cancer diagnosis and was told she had two weeks to live, and she should get all of her affairs in order. She told the doctor that she still had things to do and that she'd come back in two weeks and the cancer would be gone. The doctor thought she was crazy but the appointment for tests was made. She came back two weeks later, and the cancer was completely gone.

She shared this story with me and told me to never allow anyone to give me a diagnosis. The words she used were, "with God all things are possible," and she assured me that anything that had been created could also be uncreated. Because of this, I have never had a cancer diagnosis, nor have I feared one. Her words brought me a keen awareness that would put me on a path of discovery as an adult. This thought, implanted in my mind, made it so that I lived a life free of fear of diagnosis. When I heard fear-based news stories and diagnoses given to people I cared about, it ultimately led me to question a diagnosis instead of automatically believing what I had heard.

I have seen and heard about hundreds of people recovering from a diagnosis using alternative methods. About a year ago, as I meditated on what the next step in my journey would be, it came to me clearly that it was time for me to do whatever I could to spread this good news to the world.

WHY DO YOU THINK IT'S SO IMPORTANT FOR PEOPLE TO BE AWARE OF HOW THE BODY HEALS ITSELF?

I believe that we should always be presented with all the information available before making choices that effect our health and well-being. Repeatedly I've seen people I care about accepting a diagnosis from one conventional doctor (a specialist in a specific field of medicine) without getting a second or even a third opinion. Might there be alternative options?

For thousands of years natural remedies have been used very successfully in other countries. Many remedies now referred to as "old wives' tales" or "non-scientific quackery" existed right here in the United States before John D. Rockefeller funded the Flexner Report submitted to Congress in 1910, which vilified natural remedies in favor of the allopathic medicine he was heavily invested in.

Why are people willing to take one person's opinion without exploring all the options? Might there be a healing plan that doesn't include invasive surgery, chemotherapy, or other scary options and that doesn't take the patient right to the edge of death? This has always been something of keen interest to me. I have observed miracles happen without these options. I have heard story after story, from functional medical practitioners, of remarkable recoveries using herbs, plants, tinctures, teas, meditation, and spiritual practices, sometimes by themselves or in tandem with more conventional remedies. I believe there is more than one path to everything. And who better to make the ultimate decision regarding our health than you and me? And shouldn't we base our decisions on our own research and inner guidance system?

I want everyone to live the best and longest life possible. If I am able to bring into the light information that encourages the masses to seek and explore all possibilities, I must do so. My goal is to introduce the world to the functional medical practitioners I have met, interviewed, and learned from over the years. Our publishing company has published well over a hundred books, most of which feature cutting-edge difference makers in the fields of health and healing.

About twenty-three years ago, I created a mission statement from the question, "Why are you here, Keith?" The answer that came to me from breathing into this inquiry question was, "To touch and inspire the lives of all whom I meet." All my actions from that point on have been taken with this mission statement in mind. If one person reads this book, acts on tips and tools presented by the experts in the book, and reverses a scary diagnosis through non-conventional methods, I believe I have lived that mission.

WHAT ADVICE DO YOU HAVE FOR CREATING HEALTH AND VITALITY FROM THE INSIDE OUT?

Here are my recommendations based on what I have done to stay healthy, free of disease, and out of the hospital for most of my life:

- Eat healthy plant-based foods and take natural vitamin/mineral supplements.

- Maintain a daily spiritual practice and affirmations.

- Work out, walk, and be as active as possible.

- Explore every option before moving forward with health decisions.

- Seek many opinions from a variety of experts in different fields.

- Research all possibilities and trust your inner guidance to make the decision best for you.

- Stay away from conventional medical doctors unless in an acute trauma situation.

To date, I have had one knee surgery when I damaged my meniscus playing baseball. When I was a child, my mother took me to the emergency room for a high fever, sprained wrist, and a few stitches. Since I became old enough to make my own health journey choices, I have done my best to stay away from traditional doctors. If I have an emergency, I want a western medical doctor. If not an immediate problem, I seek many options before making my decision regarding next steps.

The few times I went to a medical doctor, they tried to give me something. One time, when a job wanted me to take a physical, I let a traditional doctor talk me into a blood test. He tried to give me some type of liver disease diagnosis. I told him what my aunt told her doctor when I was a child. I told him I would come back a few weeks later and re-test, and the appearance of the disease he was trying to give me would not be evident in the blood test.

I left, did my own process, went back a few weeks later, tested, and it was indeed gone. The doctor was befuddled. What if I had just listened to him and started taking synthetic poisonous drugs? What side effects would that have caused? Would he have then prescribed another drug to mask the side effects from the first drug he had given me? I had seen too much at that point to take his word for it. I had to try my own process — the one my aunt had inspired me with when I was in my youth.

I have had back issues for most of my life. If only my aunt had told me that what she shared with me about cancer could repair back issues as well. I say this jokingly, but truth be told, I did not put two and two together. Growing up, my mother and I worked swap meets and flea markets. As a child, I was lifting heavy boxes in and out of a station wagon. I don't remember my mother saying, "Lift with your knees, not your back." Because of this, I had what I referred to as a *bad back* at a very young age. Thanks to chiropractors, I was able to keep helping her, as they would put my back into alignment, which helped right up until the next time we worked a swap meet.

Over the years I was in several car accidents. In my late twenties a big screen TV fell on my shoulder, which was traumatic to my already sore body. It pinched a nerve in my neck, and my left arm became numb and tingly. Because the accident with the big screen happened at work, my employer forced me to see a conventional doctor. First, the doctor had me try physical therapy while encouraging pain pills. When physical therapy produced no decrease in pain, their recommendation was surgery. You've probably read enough to know I wasn't entertaining that option. Ultimately, it was a chiropractor who treated me and got the tingling and numbness to go away in my left arm and hand. However, the pain level in my upper back between my shoulders began to increase. As I continued to work jobs that had me sitting in one spot, my pain level ramped up to a level nine or ten most days.

I began to search for non-surgical methods. For this one thing, I was not able to get any results. I tried everything; chiropractors, acupuncture, Reiki, cortisone shots, pills, tinctures—you name it, I tried it. Nothing helped. I lived with chronic pain for twenty-three years. Finally I connected with two of our authors (also really good friends at this point), and they asked me what I had already tried.

First, I worked with Dr. Karen Kan. She has created a healing method of her own, and we met twice to do her process. The pain started to subside. Then I worked with Lisa Warner. I did one session on the phone with her, and then we had an in-person meeting. Lisa shared some of what she has learned about German New Medicine (now referred to Germanic Healing Knowledge) and helped me trace back to the original trauma that started my "bad back story" so long ago. She also shared how pain indicates that the body is actually healing. When I was in pain, I was always trying to do something to get rid of the pain. She shared that if I was willing to accept the pain as healing, and lean into it instead of resisting it, after a while it would subside. Then, once I thought it was over, there would be a second wave. If I was again willing to allow it instead of resisting it and get through the second wave, it would leave me. Well, I did what she taught me, and it worked. Twenty-three years of chronic pain, GONE.

The combination of working with Dr. Karen (KarenKan. com) and Lisa Warner (ConnectingYouToYou.com) had finally helped free me of a twenty-three-year chronic pain story, and I could finally begin to live a life I had never known — one free of pain.

This leads to my last piece of advice. Read each chapter in this book, identify the experts with whom you connect the most, contact them, and work with them.

About the Author

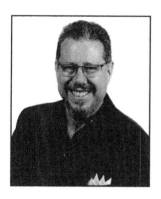

Keith Leon S. is a seven-time Award Winning, nine-time International Bestselling Author. He owns a successful publishing company, and he is a speaker/trainer who is well known as "The Book Guy."

Keith has appeared on many popular radio and television broadcasts on ABC, CBS, NBC, and *The Jenny McCarthy Show*, and his work has been covered by *Inc. Magazine*, *LA Weekly*, *The Huffington Post*, *Published Magazine*, and *Succeed Magazine*.

With his wife, Maura, Keith co-authored the book *The Seven Steps to Successful Relationships*, acclaimed by bestselling authors John Gray and Terry Cole-Whittaker. Keith is author of the bestselling books *Who Do You Think You Are? Discover the Purpose of Your Life* and *Walking with My Angels: A True Story*, both with a foreword by *Chicken Soup for the Soul* author, Jack Canfield.

Keith's publishing company has published well over one hundred books, including recent releases, *Navigating the Clickety Clack: How to Live a Peace-Filled Life in a Seemingly Toxic World* (Volumes 1, 2, 3, and 4). Keith's passion is teaching people how to go from first thought to bestseller and to create what he calls "The World's Greatest Business Card."

Find out more:

BeyondBeliefPublishing.com

LeonSmithPublishing.com

theINsideeffects.com

Maura Leon S.

WHEN AND HOW DID YOU FIRST DISCOVER THE BODY HAS THE INNATE ABILITY TO HEAL ITSELF?

I was raised in the mountains of rural Northeastern Vermont in the 1960s and 70s, my parents having moved up there from the Boston area before I was born. My mom was what was known in those days as a "health nut" because she was crazy enough to believe that feeding her family natural foods from our own garden was better than giving us the processed stuff. We were surrounded by hippies—artists, musicians, poets, teachers—all lovers of this peaceful, natural life, and I spent most of my time outdoors, walking barefoot on the ground, swimming in the brook, and climbing trees.

As I grew into young adulthood, I had little to no interest in doctors, diagnoses, or medications of any kind. I had by that point been indoctrinated, to some degree, into the standard disempowering, fear-based mainstream ideologies via the public education system, television programming, religious teachings, and the money matrix. As a result, and being the highly sensitive soul that I am, stress got the better of me, and by the time I was in my early thirties, I found myself receiving a medical diagnosis of a so-called autoimmune condition called Graves' Disease. They told me it was due to an overactive thyroid that was wreaking havoc on my body, and the only solution was radioactive iodine "therapy" to destroy most of my thyroid, thereby causing it to stop misbehaving, at which point I'd have to be on thyroid replacement medication for the rest of my life.

I told them, "Thanks, but no thanks," and set out to discover how to heal myself naturally. While it was not what I would call an easy process, I stuck with it and, eventually, it worked. The healing process encompassed physical, mental, emotional, and spiritual transformation. It was the best thing I could have done for myself.

WHY DO YOU THINK IT'S SO IMPORTANT FOR PEOPLE TO BE AWARE OF HOW THE BODY HEALS ITSELF?

Somewhere along the line, for whatever reason, we seem to have lost our way.

One day in March 2020, a friend from Los Angeles texted saying they were about to go into lockdown. What did that even mean? I had no idea, but it kinda freaked me out. The next thing I knew, we were getting similar instructions in Vermont, and I learned that it was happening all over the world. What could possibly warrant this? It made no sense to me whatsoever (and still doesn't).

I was then informed about the mandates of masking and social distancing, and I was completely horrified. Not because I believed there was actually something so horrible going around that such measures were justified, but because, again, I could not think of any justification for such an order, and all I could envision was people becoming afraid — of themselves and of each other — and being separated, divided, and controlled by a (misguided? insane? psychotic? evil?) government-media-medical establishment.

While a lot of people complied, a lot of others did not. While a lot of people believed what they were told, a lot of others did extensive research and discovered some very significant information that had been deeply hidden for a very long time.

As excruciating as this whole ordeal has been — and continues to be — to get through, it appears to be a very important experience for our collective consciousness to process. In my view, our future depends upon our individual realization of who and what we really are. We are creators. We are not victims of circumstances; we create our circumstances. Our bodies are not fragile and vulnerable; they are brilliant, dynamic, self-regulating, vibrational powerhouses.

It's time to take our power back. To varying degrees individually, we gave it away and pretended to be victims, convinced that we were at war with our own bodies, with other living beings, and with the earth. We are not, and we have no need to be. The power of love heals all wounds. The power of peace allows all of life to flow in perfect harmony. We have that power. We just need to use it.

To me, it appears that the events of these past few years are showing us that only when we have freed our minds of the concept of disease can we create a future of peace and prosperity.

WHAT ADVICE DO YOU HAVE FOR CREATING HEALTH AND VITALITY FROM THE INSIDE OUT?

Most of our problems are all in our heads. So the first thing to do is to stop believing your thoughts, particularly when they are not peaceful, productive thoughts. It's okay if the thoughts come into your mind; just don't feed them, entertain them, and invite them to stay.

Find the ways that work for you to relax your mind. Allow yourself to become peaceful. Focus on your heart. Think about love and gratitude. Focus on the people you love. Do something nice for them. It's really very simple. Don't overcomplicate it.

Once your mind is relaxed, you can start to tune in to what your body is telling you. It's telling you everything you need to know about how to get out of its way so it can do what it was designed to do: be strong and healthy for you. You don't need to fix it. It will fix itself. You just have to stop getting in the way.

Again, it is really that simple. Stop overcomplicating it and let it be easy.

The more you relax your mind and tune in to your body, the more you will learn to trust your intuition. You will be amazed at your ability to know what to do and when and how to do it. Just like a muscle, your intuition will get stronger and stronger the more you use it. That's all it is — a simple regular practice of noticing what your inner guidance is telling you, and then noticing what happens when you follow it and what happens when you don't follow it. Just keep doing that and collecting data. Soon, you'll realize your true power. Your body will support you. Your life will support you. And others will begin to notice and be inspired by you.

You can do this. I didn't believe I could at first, but then I decided to give it a try anyway, because the alternative was not peaceful, and I wanted a life of peace. So, I experimented with it. The more I did, the more I began to trust it, and the more I trusted it, the better it worked. It's like a "vicious cycle" but, instead, it's a delicious cycle!

Stop believing all the negative, fear-based crapola, and start believing in yourself and your ability to heal and to thrive. And you will! Especially when you surround yourself with positive, peaceful, productive people. That's what I recommend.

About the Author

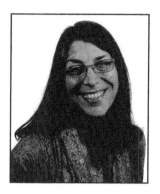

Maura Leon S. is an inspirational publisher and author, intuitive life coach, and vibrational artist. Her Vibrational Visioning process has been praised by transformational leaders, including best-selling authors Marci Shimoff and Maribel Jimenez.

In 1999, Maura succeeded in manifesting the relationship of her dreams, using a specific process to attract exactly what she wanted. She then discovered that her soulmate, Keith, had used the exact same process to attract her. Realizing that they had a common mission, Keith and Maura wrote and published their first book, *The Seven Steps to Successful Relationships: A Practical Guide for Everyone,* and began teaching people how to communicate better, love themselves more completely, and make their dream lives a reality.

In 2012, Maura was a contributing author in the book, *You Make a Difference: 50 Heart-Centered Entrepreneurs Share Their Stories of Inspiration and Transformation.*

In 2015, Keith and Maura developed the YouSpeakIt book program to make it easy, fast, and affordable for busy entrepreneurs and leading-edge health practitioners to get their mission and message out to the world. In this program, authors can speak their book in just seven phone calls.

Maura is co-owner of Babypie Publishing and is Keith Leon S.'s biggest fan and supporter.

Find out more at: LeonSmithPublishing.com and BeyondBeliefPublishing.com.

Trisha Schmalhofer

WHEN AND HOW DID YOU FIRST DISCOVER THE BODY HAS THE INNATE ABILITY TO HEAL ITSELF?

As a child I knew that prescription medicines were not the answer because whenever I did get sick, which was rare, and Mom got a prescription from the doctor, I would take one or two, it made me feel weird, and I would stop taking it. What ended up helping me heal was time, rest, fresh air, sunshine, and some home remedies like chicken corn soup, warm washcloths on my head, and Mom's love. I now know that the weird feeling was my intuition guiding me and my body signaling that the pill was not a good match.

When I was twenty-five, I had an inner calling to switch careers and explore massage therapy and various types of alternative medicine. I studied craniosacral therapy, which is a subtle yet deep touch therapy that works with the inner physician (IP)—the innate, connected, all-knowing part of us that directs the healing processes of the body, mind, and spirit. In my experience, the IP communicates to us through the fascia (connective tissue web) with rhythms, pulses, unwinding tissue, heat exchange, and energy waves.

The inner physician also communicates through our extra sensory perception of clairaudience (hearing in your mind), clairsentience (feeling in your being), claircognizance (knowing in your gut), clairvoyance (seeing in your mind), and clairtangency (seeing/feeling with your hands). Every person can communicate in these subtle ways. One or two perceptions tend to be stronger and are used every day, sometimes without even being conscious of it.

During healing work, the client's inner physician leads the session, and my role is to listen, facilitate, support, and witness the miracles that take place. It is important that people are aware they have an inner physician connected to *all* parts of themselves. Awareness is the first step in all healing pathways. Every day I teach people how to sense and listen to their own IP in their authentic way to facilitate their own healing.

Why do you think it's so important for people to be aware of how the body heals itself?

We are sovereign beings who have free will. When you believe your body knows exactly how to heal itself and your role is to listen and support it, it gives you the freedom many of us are seeking. You can choose what to put into your body to support its healing. You can choose the type of movement and expression that will assist you in healthy cellular and tissue repair, fluid flow, and energy distribution. Your body is designed to ebb and flow, expand and contract. It keeps you alive, strives for homeostasis, and performs optimally based on what is taken in and released. You have the privilege to choose your food, supplements, information, energy, environmental influences, thoughts, beliefs, and attitude. You are a complex system that is designed to be adaptable and resilient, and every system and organ knows its job. You have the power to give the body the resources it needs to be the healthiest it can possibly be.

When you have pain, pressure, or numbness, the body is communicating that it's stuck and needs support or it's in a natural healing process. It may be talking softly with a gentle nudge, or it can be screaming. Your body is always in a state of movement, shifting, re-apportioning, re-balancing. Educating yourself about anatomy and physiology can help you understand your body's language. Receiving treatments from wholistic-minded health practitioners can help you connect to your body and support your healing process. Understanding that emotions are stored in the body and exploring ways to move the feelings through will also be empowering and help transform you into a more balanced, healthy person.

One of my recent personal health challenges was uterine fibroids. These are masses of tissue that build up in the uterus and can cause pain and limit function of surrounding organs. They never caused a problem for me until one of them doubled in size in three years. I supported my healing by going into meditation and dialoguing with the fibroids, and they told me they were saving my life by storing toxins. To support my body's healing, I changed my diet and took natural supplements for detoxification, dissolving the excess tissue, and balancing my hormones. I devoted myself to a daily practice with qigong, dancing, breathwork, prayer, sound therapy, guided meditation, tantra, yoga, and walking outdoors. I practiced shamanic journeying to receive guidance and love from Spirit. I received healing and prayer from friends, family, massage therapists, shamans, Christians, pagans, acupuncturists, energy medicine practitioners, and mediums. I committed to a nine-month structured program that taught the Taoist ancient wisdom approach called Living Sexology. Within a year, the fibroids significantly shrank in size, and they continue to dissolve. My body told me what it needed. I simply had to ask and listen.

WHAT ADVICE DO YOU HAVE FOR CREATING HEALTH AND VITALITY FROM THE INSIDE OUT?

Keep an open mind that is curious and teachable. Listen to new perspectives, try new experiences, receive help from trusted therapists and facilitators to work through the shadow parts of yourself, and then discern what is truth to you. Take what resonates and leave the rest. If you walk through life with a closed mind, focused on narrow, toxic experiences, or perceived trauma, you're limiting yourself and inhibiting your growth and healing. It is important to have a childlike mind — like being on an adventure. Be curious, seek knowledge, seek growth opportunities, deepen your connection to yourself at the core, and expand your wisdom.

It is important to ask and receive the guidance and to receive the guidance in your own way. You may ask questions like: *What do I need to add or take away to feel excited about my life? What emotion may be contributing to this rash I am getting on my face?* Listen to nature, listen to your body, listen to books, and listen to other people talk about their experiences or share their wisdom, especially vibrant elders. In our culture today we do not listen to our elders enough. They have gems of wisdom that come out when we slow down and are in a quiet space with them. When you get through the surface stuff and sink in deep with them, that's when the medicine comes. You receive something you need that causes a "quickening" in your being, a vibration of change that starts deep in the cells. This can cause a spontaneous healing in your body or an *ah ha* in your mind. You can also receive this type of medicine when you sit in play space with children and enter their world of innocent questioning and rapid learning.

Devote yourself to a daily practice or routine that aligns all parts of you — mind, body, spirit, soul, emotions, and beyond. You are a multidimensional being with many contributing factors to physical symptoms that are emerging. Meditation or mindfulness practices in any form that cultivate a role of observer is essential for healing. This helps you get into a state of mind to listen and receive without getting caught up in stressful thinking or emotional overwhelm. Regular movement that you enjoy is also an important part of your daily practice. Moving with intention can alchemize emotions and turn unfavorable feelings like anger and sorrow into waves of healing elixirs flowing through the body. Emotions are simply waves of energy that are interpreted by the brain as good or bad. Energy can be transformed through intention, breath, and movement.

Regularly spending time in nature helps you connect more deeply in a spiritual way. Being around people who uplift and cultivate happiness is also important to create health and vitality. Devoting yourself to a daily practice helps you feel centered in your core; feel gratitude more easily; visualize your body healing more clearly; communicate with your parts more directly; distribute your energy; and direct your organs, cells, and tissues to heal with ease and grace.

About the Author

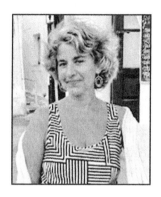

Trisha Schmalhofer (aka SoulFire) is a whisperer of the body, alchemist of the spirit, and channel for divine wisdom. She has a knack for helping beings of all ages to feel comfortable in this Earth experience by deeply listening on all levels and guiding them through transformation to balance. Trisha has been licensed in craniosacral therapy, SomatoEmotional Release, and various types of massage for over twenty-six years, and she opened her private MedHealers practice in 2016. She is certified in Systems Informed Therapy, Soul Realignment akashic records access, and energy and sound therapy, and she is a professional intuitive, sage, and frequency medicine woman.

Trisha has a love for percussion and creates her own soundscapes—featuring gong, drum, rattle, bells, voice, and nature sounds. She plays on stage with various musicians and the group Mystic Sounds.

In 2019, Trisha felt the call to build a personal and spiritual growth community named BAM: Badasses, Alchemists, Mystics. Trisha guides you in single sessions or groups to access your own Inner Healer, clear the pathway for your Core Essence to emerge from within, and trust yourself to discern as you navigate the waves of the world. She is available in Florida or to travel to you for retreats, multi-day sessions, and intimate small group intensives. Trisha also has an extensive virtual practice to accommodate her international clientele.

If you feel drawn to Trisha and sense she may help you through your current spiritual transformation, energy/emotional block, or healing phase you are journeying through, email: medhealersinfo@gmail.com or go to medhealers.com to schedule a complimentary clarity call. To view the BAM events, lives and podcasts, go to bamcommunity11.com.

Sharla Lee Shults

WHEN AND HOW DID YOU FIRST DISCOVER THE BODY HAS THE INNATE ABILITY TO HEAL ITSELF?

As a child, we all learn from cuts, bruises, and skinned knees that the body has a miraculous way of healing itself. Even fractured and broken bones mend and regain their strength. Do we question or research why or how this occurs? Rarely, if ever. It is accepted. It just happens and is seldom connected to daily health and well-being.

The flip side of this automatic healing process lies in how we view ourselves, which governs our actions/reactions and overall fitness. One look in the mirror incites prejudgment. Are you familiar with the metaphor *you are what you eat?* This sparks a serious question, one that goes deeper than simply examining the foods you are eating. The question becomes, "Have you given serious thought to what you are feeding your cells, the basic units of life?" Physical, mental, emotional, and spiritual well-being are dependent upon healthy cells.

In other words, the body functions from the inside out, rather than outside in.

In 2017, my husband passed away after an extended illness. We were together for nearly thirty-three years. From 2017 to 2019, my mental and physical capacities suffered, which greatly affected me emotionally and spiritually. What I saw of myself on a daily basis only mirrored the outside appearance, neglecting my inside battle for life. I literally became a recluse until I traveled to visit my daughter, Nicole, in North Carolina in December 2019.

My first eye-opener was how exhausted I felt by simply getting up the stairs to the front door. I huffed and puffed, grabbing the handrails with each step, stopping to catch my breath when I reached the platform at the top of the stairs. Then when I opened the door, I gasped! In front of me were additional stairways, one down to the level where I would be sleeping and another up to the kitchen. I almost went into panic mode. I would have to climb two sets of stairs between my bedroom and the kitchen numerous times each day. I could go outside from the downstairs den but to venture into the wooded area in front of the house, I faced the initial stairs again and the repeated stairways to my bedroom and the kitchen. The alternative: become a recluse downstairs.

I was emaciated and weak due to an improper diet, insufficient hydration, and lack of exercise. This could be compared to persons with anorexia who see themselves as being normal or overweight, when actually, they are the complete opposite.

I endured pain from the moment I arose in the morning until retiring for the night but had learned to live with it. That was acceptance as a result of my life's change. All the while, my body's cells were crying out, but my own lack of awareness dismantled my capacity to listen.

In rapid succession, like a flash camera snapping pictures, my mind began to spark thoughts of doctors' visits, examinations, blood tests, x-rays, other forms of testing, and medical bills. My daughter enlightened me with a different approach. With a series of questions, Nicole analyzed my daily routine — lack of restful sleep, one meal a day, and maybe drinking eight ounces of water which is hardly enough to survive. The high-powered sleeping pills I was taking only made me more lethargic. My daily exercise consisted of walking from one room to another.

I could choose to remain in a state of poor health, visiting doctors frequently, seeking temporary "feel good" medications, or I could accept the need for change and learn to listen to my body. Doctor visits and pills would only feed my problems, whereas listening to my body would open the door to better health by nourishing the cells from within.

Accepting what needed to change and putting those changes into action would be a challenge. What did I have to lose? My life if I did not listen to my body. What would I gain? My life as a fluently flowing stream, rather than one battling turbulent waters!

As I began my journey back to good health, my focus shifted from concentrating on everything that was wrong with me to understanding what my body was telling me. I examined good health at the cellular level, boosting the cells' natural healing processes with nutritional shakes instead of taking pills to mask my symptoms. I learned to use kinesiology as a biofeedback tool that led me to making healthier choices and exercising better decisions.

That is also when I discovered the healing powers and absolute joy of Mother Nature. It doesn't require a long journey into the realm of nature. It can be as simple as looking out your kitchen window or stepping outside into your own backyard. The body reacts positively to the natural environment, replacing stress with relaxation. I stepped beyond the box, leaving familiarity behind for new territory, and created a true bond.

After only two weeks of integrating the rejuvenation and healing process within my body, I awoke feeling like a new person. I bounded out of bed, tackling both sets of stairs like a gazelle running from its prey. Upon landing at the top of the stairs leading into the kitchen, I raised my arms in victory like Rocky Balboa in Philadelphia! My daughter and son-in-law will attest to this!

Today, my mind is sharper. I am no longer an emotional wreck. My physical activity begins at sunrise with an early morning walk. I step away from the busyness and business of daily strife into the comforting and healing spirit of Mother Nature. Taking 10,000 steps a day is easy, and it's not unusual for the miles to reach five or more. I thank my body, and every cell of my body thanks me each day in return.

Through my daily walks, I solidified that one of the best healing atmospheres is the natural world. Mother Nature arouses enhanced realization of our planet Earth, along with her vital role. Within nature, I discover places of exhilaration and gateways to understanding, along with exposure to a world of contentment. These in themselves relieve stress and anxiety, allowing the natural healing processes of the body to do their job.

WHY DO YOU THINK IT'S SO IMPORTANT FOR PEOPLE TO BE AWARE OF HOW THE BODY HEALS ITSELF?

Awareness of how your body works brings into focus the areas of balance and nutrition, rather than getting on the fast track to see doctors and taking medications whose side effects can be harmful. Balance and nutrition can be improved by assisting the body in its natural healing processes, which begin with the cells inside the body. This promotes attention to a longer and healthier life.

My intention is not to degrade the role of doctors and nurses, nor the need for medications when duly warranted. Awareness allows concentration to be placed on your body's signs from the onset of the appearance or feeling something may be wrong.

I was unaware of my declining health because I had focused solely on the drastic change in my life when my husband passed away. Health considerations were on the back burner, barely simmering. It took someone else, my daughter, to recognize the downhill spiral I was in to lead me to working from the inside out. Having awareness of the body and mind at the cellular level takes on a totally new perspective.

WHAT ADVICE DO YOU HAVE FOR CREATING HEALTH AND VITALITY FROM THE INSIDE OUT?

Listen to *your* body. It talks to you with symptoms. You can dwell on the symptom making it worse, or you can accept the symptom as a signal something needs to change.

You may be thinking, "So, I accept it. Now what?" The answer is simple, "Take action!"

Begin with simple changes in daily routine. If you don't have a healthy routine, develop one. This will foster your body's ability to heal itself. Remain conscious of your daily nutrition and hydration. Add to this, daily walks in nature that provide an optimal healing environment. Inhale deeply and hold on to the healing spirit from within. Exhale slowly!

Mindfulness of what is going on inside your body allows you to increase your awareness of functions that are out of order. Know your body. Pay attention. Know *your* signs, for each person is their own individual. The more attention you pay to your internal being instead of your external being, the quicker you will heal from the inside out.

It's a win-win when you let the inside healing begin! Beginning the healing process from within eases discomfort both inside and outside, rather than placing a shining light on the dis-ease. The key is to recognize the signs when the body is out of sync. Step back and listen intently as the body speaks its language of healing. I will celebrate my seventy-seventh birthday in September 2023, living the life I love without prescription drugs. That in itself is a milestone to be proud of! Happy trails, my friends! I await the next sunrise and new writing adventures.

Life is fragile. Treasure it! Nature is bountiful. Notice it! Awareness leads to action.

See it. . . hear it. . . feel it! Let the healing begin from within!

About the Author

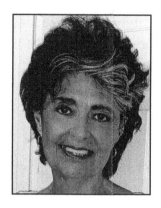

Sharla Lee Shults graduated from Troy University (Alabama). She began teaching high school chemistry and mathematics, then a move to Ohio led her to the middle school classroom. Four years later, she ventured outside education into the railroad industry in Panama City, Florida.

Sharla reentered education after an eleven-year break. Experiences from her railroad career provided real-world connections to the classroom. She worked with Special Olympics and was instrumental in establishing Exchange Club youth organizations in three Panama City high schools. Sharla's last classroom experiences involved working with teens in an at-risk dropout prevention program. While involved in this endeavor, she introduced a Poetic Math Challenge, which uncovered her passion as a poetic mathematician.

In 2001, Sharla left the classroom but remained in the field of education with Beacon Educator in the Bay District School System, writing curriculum and providing professional development for teachers across the state of Florida. She semiretired in 2008, at which time she became an Online Learning Specialist for Beacon.

Sharla's latest book is *Catnip of Life*, released in March 2023. This collection of poetry is the gateway to understanding Mother Nature's footprints.

Her other publications include *Echoes* (2004), *Remembering* (2009), and *Awakenings* (2012). Watch for her upcoming books: *A Touch of Catnip, Voices in Nature,* and *Buzzin'*, a children's title.

Her website catnipoflife.info and blog catnipoflife.com offer awareness boosters of the world around you. Contact her for more information at poetrybysharla@gmail.com.

JP Sears

WHEN AND HOW DID YOU FIRST DISCOVER THE BODY HAS THE INNATE ABILITY TO HEAL ITSELF?

In July 2001 I was twenty years old. I will never forget; I was taking a class with my first mentor, Paul Check, a powerful human being who is still a great friend. I thought I was taking a class on exercise science, which I was, but it was also a lot more than that. In the class I learned a lot of body pain is caused by emotions. That just blew my mind. I was intrigued. I was fascinated. It was like, *wow, the world is not what I thought it was. I am not what I thought I was.* I learned that body pain — back pain, shoulder pain, neck pain — can be caused by emotions; specifically, unexpressed emotions that are trapped in the body.

That was a profound day for me back in July 2001. It has changed the whole trajectory of how I look at myself, take care of my health, and try to influence those around me. Paul Check also taught me about the chakra system and how specific emotional issues will influence positive or negative regions of the body based on the chakra system coloration. That was a powerful experience for me. That was my entry point and, of course, I have gone deeper since then. That is when I started to learn how the inner life — our emotions, our mind, our spirit — influences what we call our physical health. But, spoiler alert, I now call our physical health mostly just a symptom of what is going on in our minds, emotions, and our relationship with our soul.

WHY DO YOU THINK IT'S SO IMPORTANT FOR PEOPLE TO BE AWARE OF HOW THE BODY HEALS ITSELF?

It is important for people to be aware of how the body heals itself because it is *their* body. I believe people deserve to know how their bodies work. It is kind of like when you buy a car, it comes with an owner's manual. You deserve to have the owner's manual. You deserve to understand how the car functions because it is *your* car.

We are incarnated in these beautiful bodies. It is a miraculous gift, and I firmly believe we are not only empowered but, of course, I think we need to have the right to know how our bodies operate. I believe that health equals freedom. I think freedom is a gift from God. I think it is our natural state of being. However, no matter how constitutional someone is, and they might be frolicking in green pastures of the freest country on earth but if they do not have their health, they are not a free individual.

There are some negative influences in our world that work to distract people and keep them unaware of the basic ancient knowledge of how our bodies actually heal. When a person knows how their body heals and how it thrives, they are incredibly empowered. But I believe there are some people in our world who probably were not held enough as children, who have become invested in trying to control other people. It is hard to control empowered people. But it is pretty easy to control disempowered people, especially in the form of sickness if they are not feeling well, if they have things going in their body, their brain, and their emotions or are suffering from depression. It is very easy to control them. Unfortunately, people get controlled at the expense of themselves. They are fed, I would call it, propaganda. "Hey, if you are sick, then the path to wellness is down this pharmaceutical aisle." People deserve better than that.

People certainly deserve to have the option of any sort of pharmaceutical route that they deem to be in their best interest. But I do think that there is a deliberate attempt to disconnect people from the miraculous healing abilities of their own body and mind, which occur if things are just put in place that need to be put in place. It is essential that people have their birthright of freedom, which necessitates they have their health. To maintain their health, they have to have a pretty basic knowledge of what the body needs to heal.

WHAT ADVICE DO YOU HAVE FOR CREATING HEALTH AND VITALITY FROM THE INSIDE OUT?

Take small steps. A big mistake people can make in trying to create health and vitality from the inside out is they see where they are, envision where they want to be, then try to get there all at once. It is almost a futile effort. Nobody can run a marathon in one stride. The path to great vitality and health is usually built by doing small things very consistently. One of the most important pieces of advice I would offer is see where you are, see where you want to go, and then establish the next step for you based on where you are at that moment. Then when you take that step, cherish it. Treat that step with reverence. Become consistent with it and then take the next step. Rather than trying to take a whole mile-long stride, which is just a recipe for failure, take one step at a time.

It is really important to think in three hundred sixty degrees with your health and vitality from the inside out. What I mean by that is acknowledge the full spectrum of possibilities. Work on your emotions. Work on your purpose. Become more aligned with those. Work on your nutrition. Work on your lifestyle. Work on deciding which specific supplements are right for you. Work on your stress reduction. I know that can sound overwhelming, like, "Well, JP you just said take one small step at a time and now you are saying address the whole three hundred sixty degrees."

No. When you are establishing what the next steps are, at least for me, I tend to avoid addressing the uncomfortable areas. I find it very comfortable to make strides in my nutrition, my exercise, even my lifestyle practices. It is more challenging for me to make strides in my emotional well-being and healing emotional issues I may have carried for a very long time — letting go of resentments, letting go of shame — working on that.

When you are looking at creating health from the inside out, you need to think in a holistic three hundred sixty degree lens and not be tempted to just do the easier parts. Typically, the parts you *do not* want to address are the parts you need to address the most.

Ask for help. There are so many resources out there — professionals, authors, online videos, a lot of legitimate helpful advice. The experts can save you time and years of trial and error. I personally do a lot of consulting with experts, working with them one on one so I can accelerate my healing and vitality journey. Reach out to save yourself time, energy, and pain. Accept help from people who have knowledge in the areas of inner health.

And with that I would also say it is always important to own the self-responsibility of steering your own ship. Consult with your inner physician, the guidance of your heart, what makes sense to your own critical thinking, and always let that be the main compass you use to navigate your decisions and next steps.

About the Author

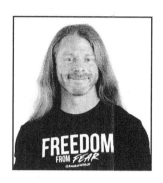

JP Sears is a YouTuber, comedian, author, and speaker, and a curious student of life. His work takes an unapologetic stand for freedom, free speech, and encouraging people to live free from fear. His content has served over seven million followers and acquired 600 million views. When JP's not making videos or performing on stage, he loves to spend time at home with his family in the great state of Texas.

Find out more:

awakenwithjp.com/
instagram.com/awakenwithjp
facebook.com/awakenwithjp
youtube.com/awakenwithjp
twitter.com/awakenwithjp

Dr. Elizabeth Hesse Sheehan, DC PscD

WHEN AND HOW DID YOU FIRST DISCOVER THE BODY HAS THE INNATE ABILITY TO HEAL ITSELF?

When I was sixteen years old, I was in a car accident. I sustained several injuries, including a concussion, whiplash, temporomandibular joint dysfunction (TMJ), and severe soft tissue and joint injury to my spine that resulted in chronic fatigue, chronic pain syndrome, and other issues that impacted my life for six years. After going through many mainstream doctors, it was the chiropractors who taught me about the Innate Intelligence of the body and who ultimately helped me. That experience inspired me to become a chiropractor and help empower people to heal without drugs or surgery.

WHY DO YOU THINK IT'S SO IMPORTANT FOR PEOPLE TO BE AWARE OF HOW THE BODY HEALS ITSELF?

Allopathic medicine is the third leading cause of death in the United States. The events of the last three years may have pushed that number to the second or first place spot, as we see the rise in excess deaths.

We live in a culture heavily reliant on giving our power away. We have been conditioned to believe that health is determined by fate or genetics. It is normal for people of all ages to be on multiple pharmaceutical interventions. We are taught to pop a pill to alleviate our symptoms, versus looking at the underlying root causes of our symptoms and addressing them at that level. This is akin to taking the batteries out of your smoke detector instead of putting out the fire! When you look at the causes of death, from largely preventable factors like heart disease and cancer, this is definitely a fire!

We are no longer taught the truth about the basic foundational practices that create health and vitality. These include a healthy diet from whole organic foods; hydration with clean water; getting sunlight, fresh air, exercise, and electromagnetic field (EMF) mitigation; sleep hygiene practices, and stress management. Detoxification strategies are vital, as is reconnecting to nature.

Despite all of these factors, it is important to *know* you can heal!

Your body is a self-healing organism. This is one of the foundational teachings of vitalistic philosophy. The body can heal itself, providing things are not blocking its ability to do so. Healing is orchestrated by your body's Innate Intelligence. If you cut yourself, you do not have to consciously mobilize immune cells to the area, release pain chemicals, or modulate blood flow. Your body does all that for you. That is your Innate Intelligence.

When you realize your body has an immense capacity for healing, you are empowered. Yes, it also requires a level of self-discipline and responsibility. You can work with your body, make better choices, and know that your wellness is not set in stone. Your health is not a result of fate or chance but of faith and choice.

In my twenty-three-year career as a wholistic health care provider, I have seen time and time again the body's tremendous ability to get better, to heal. I have seen people beat all the odds and, of course, I've heard the infamous "Well, you must have been misdiagnosed" when people recover from "incurable illnesses."

It is vital to know you can get better. Never let anyone tell you otherwise!

Nowhere do I see this more clearly than in my work with children and adults with Down syndrome. Two weeks after my son was born, we found out he has Down syndrome, a genetic "disorder" where there are three copies of Chromosome 21 instead of the usual two. This extra chromosome has a full complement of fully functioning genes on it—genes that very much influence the rest of the genome and the biochemistry of the body, resulting in a laundry list of different "disorders" and challenges.

Unfortunately, in our society, the prevailing thought is that Down syndrome is a horrible disease. Parents who hear this diagnosis for their child are often traumatized. The medical profession largely acts like it is worse than a death sentence, either refusing to meet the eyes of the parents or launching into a list of things they predict your child will never be able to do. This is all patently false. No one knows anyone's future.

Parents who get a prenatal diagnosis are heavily pressured to abort. Time and time again abortion will be offered, even after parents have made it known to their doctors that they love their child and abortion is not an option. Unfortunately, this pressure is so successful that approximately sixty-five percent of all babies with Down syndrome in the United States are aborted.

For years we have been trained by the mainstream to believe that if something is genetic, there is nothing we can do about it. We now know that epigenetics, those factors that control how genes express (diet, lifestyle, etc.) are also as big if not even more of a factor than the genes themselves. But when you have a child diagnosed with a genetic disorder, not just a gene mutation, this really puts things to the test.

My philosophy was challenged from the get-go with Connor's diagnosis. In addition to Down syndrome, he was born with a type of preleukemia only found in Down syndrome children, called transient myeloproliferative disorder. From that diagnosis we found out about his Down syndrome. We were thrust into the allopathic world of oncologists, cardiologists (my son had open heart surgery at three months old), and other specialists.

What is one to do when faced with an "incurable genetic disorder"?

Well, I did what I do! I used nutrition, herbs and supplements, homeopathy, essential oils, light therapy, chiropractic and other body work, and energy healing techniques. And Connor defied all the odds. He not only survived until his surgery, but he also thrived and healed quickly. The cancer went into remission on its own. To this day Connor is a very healthy, bright kid, challenging what was supposed to be.

Nowhere has it become more apparent to me that the body has a tremendous capacity to heal than working with people who have Down syndrome. For the most part, they are a very medically underserved community. Parents are often told that their child's issues are "just Down syndrome and there is nothing that can be done" when, in fact, there are diagnosable issues that deserve and require treatment. When you work within a profession that is often written off, it opens the door to so much more possibility.

I specialize in combining functional and alternative approaches with energy testing (muscle testing), and I create customized programs for each patient. I work on hacking the deviations in their biochemistry, not to change them or try to make them not have Down syndrome, for I feel strongly it is by God's design that these people have Down syndrome, and this diagnosis carries with it extraordinary gifts. By supporting the parts of biochemistry we have access to, they are able to have more support at their physical and biochemical level.

We should all be doing things to actively improve our health. I have witnessed countless dramatic transformations of the health and well-being of my patients. This, in turn, allows them to have more energy available to live out their soul's mission and their life purpose. Being able to give parents hope and tangible results is very rewarding, and it teaches all of us about the power of our own innate healing ability.

WHAT ADVICE DO YOU HAVE FOR CREATING HEALTH AND VITALITY FROM THE INSIDE OUT?

Creating health and vitality is a multi-factored process. You are more than just your physical body and biochemistry. True health must be cared for at the physical, mental, emotional, energetic, and spiritual levels. Body-mind-spirit.

Caring for yourself by including mind and spirit has direct and indirect effects on your physical health. Wholistic practitioners know that imbalances in other areas are contributing factors to the challenges your physical body faces. Many things in the physical body cannot shift until other areas are also addressed. This is something rarely addressed by mainstream medical practitioners.

People are beginning to remember ancient wisdom, and different branches of science can validate what cultures knew generations ago. One of the most impactful ways you can create health and vitality from the inside out is through energy healing.

Energy healing/energy medicine is a term used to describe various practices that work on the energy fields of the body. Energy healing has an amazingly large breadth of applications. The common goal is to help create balance within all aspects of your being, further supporting your body's ability to heal itself.

This can be done by removing blocks or interference in your body by working on meridians, chakras, and unprocessed emotions in your body, as well as sending energy in different forms to your body.

Examples of energy healing include acupuncture, reflexology, homeopathy, tapping, and light therapy. It can also involve using different frequencies and vibrations through sound, color, and intentions. Energy healing helps heal your body-mind-spirit from stresses, imbalances, and traumas.

Many people who have challenges like chronic fatigue, chronic pain syndromes, autoimmune issues, neurological issues, or ADHD are very energetically sensitive. We see this almost universally in kids with special needs like Down syndrome. If you or your child is someone who seems to pick up on the energy of a room, can feel others' pain or emotions, or is affected by unknown/unseen influences, that is energetic sensitivity. Energy healing practices are a vital tool to help balance your sensitivity and help your gifts become the blessing they are meant to be.

The beautiful thing about energy healing is that it is easy for people to learn and use with themselves and others. There are so many different techniques that everyone can find at least one way that helps them find relief.

My passion is to teach others how easy energy healing is. Children are especially receptive and open to energy healing techniques and pick them up quickly. Imagine being empowered as a child with easy ways to support yourself or to help anyone and anything. This is what the world needs more of right now! If you are reading this book, you are one of the conscious, creative, and caring souls here to help the healing of the planet!

About the Author

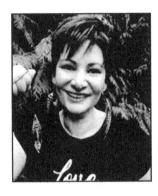

Dr. Elizabeth Hesse Sheehan is a wholistic chiropractor and nutritionist who works with her Pastoral Science and Medicine credentials in the realms of energetic healing. With a strong focus on chronic mystery illnesses and children with special needs, a big emphasis in her practice is teaching. Dr. Elizabeth's mission is to support others to unleash their inner healer, allowing the body to reach its full potential of health and vitality on all levels. Dr. Elizabeth brings over two decades of experience with a wide and eclectic array of healing modalities, including Autonomic Response Testing, Quantum Neurology, Wholistic Methylation, and natural medicine, including essential oils, crystals, and flower essences. She works with radionics and other quantum field energy modalities, Pendulum Alchemy, phototherapy, emotional release/healing modalities,

Family Constellation Therapy, and numerous kinesiology techniques.

Dr. Elizabeth has written several energy healing protocols that she teaches through her site easyenergyhealing. info, along with other courses. Her passions include homeschooling her children, serving as VP Challenger for her local Little League, and helping children with disabilities play adaptive baseball.

To learn more about how to quickly and effectively use energy healing techniques, please visit easyenergyhealing.info. Sign up for the free ebook *Easy Energy Healing.* You can also join one of Dr. Elizabeth's group sessions, sign up for one-on-one sessions, or take energy healing courses.

Dr. Odette Suter

WHEN AND HOW DID YOU FIRST DISCOVER THE BODY HAS THE INNATE ABILITY TO HEAL ITSELF?

I was in my second year of veterinary school. We had just gone through the anatomy course on horses' hooves when just a few days later, a friend from the barn I was riding at asked me if I had heard that a veterinarian from Germany was going to do a workshop about hooves in my hometown. "Do you want to go?" she inquired.

I thought to myself, *I already know everything I need to know about hooves but hey, since this is just ten minutes from home, I may as well go and find out what this is all about.* So I went, and well, life was never the same. I was forever changed because I learned not just about hooves but basically about taking horses back into as much of their natural state and lifestyle as possible, because that's the only way they can be healthy.

I had grown up horseback riding and all of those horses were stuck in a twelve-by-twelve-foot stall, kind of like a prison, with not a whole lot of exercise, just standing around. All of them were wearing iron shoes and I thought that was just normal. I was taught that riding them for an hour and then sticking them back in their stall was how horses were supposed to live.

Learning from this veterinarian blew my mind and made so much sense. *Duh and Why didn't I think of this?* is really all I could think. It had never occurred to me that they were getting sick because their lifestyle was the opposite of what nature designed for them. We remove them from their natural ways, and they become sick.

That weekend workshop was a huge eye-opener when I learned that when we go back to nature and imitate what nature provides to the body, it has the ability to heal itself. That realization carried me through vet school like a bright light of hope and possibilities. Even now, I'm in awe of what nature is capable of doing and how little we really know. Truth be told, nature doesn't need our help.

Just think about it: We have one hundred trillion cells. We have nine billion chemical reactions happening every second. We have one hundred trillion microbes in the body, and there are tens of thousands of species of microbes that live in and around us. There are trees, plants, birds, insects, the sun, day, night. We are part of an ecosystem, and that ecosystem is so complex that it would be ridiculous to think we can outsmart it or improve on it. That is where the innate ability comes from. It is from that well-designed system that is already present and has developed and evolved over billions of years.

WHY DO YOU THINK IT'S SO IMPORTANT FOR PEOPLE TO BE AWARE OF HOW THE BODY HEALS ITSELF?

We live in a culture where we have become extremely dependent on the medical establishment. We rely on other people telling us what we need to do, and we relinquish our own power, our own innate wisdom and ability to be in tune with our bodies and with nature. We give up the sense that we already know what we need.

Children and animals are extremely good at knowing what they need. Take for instance dogs who eat poop. If we observe closely, we may notice that they will only eat poop from a certain animal while completely ignoring others. They are in tune with their own bodies, and they are very much capable of discerning whether poop from a particular animal has in it what they need. I'm not suggesting that we all start eating poop—though many species will engage in coprophagy naturally when needed—but we have forgotten to listen to and trust our innate wisdom.

It is important that we open ourselves back up to that wisdom because the body already knows how to heal itself. We are highly complex beings who have evolved over a long period of time. To be able to heal again and to be aware of that innate power, we need to trust that our bodies and the entire ecosystem of this planet are refined and perfected to allow us all to thrive. There are many mechanisms that support the body's healing and its ability to resolve dis-ease and malfunctioning. If we think about how many cells we have and how many biochemical processes are going on, we can see that there are many things that could go wrong, and yet our bodies don't just fall apart at the slightest breeze. In spite of the mess we've created on this planet—the toxicity, the pollution, the abuse—our bodies are still functioning really, really well!

Why is that? It's because of that innate ability to heal. People need to be aware of this amazing power to heal, because this realization, this re-discovery of profound truth carries hope and excitement that things can turn around, and that we can take our power back and heal. Instead of just following others we become our own leaders and healers and reconnect with our leader and healer within. This way, we step out of survival mode, access our innate internal wisdom and healing, and ultimately connect with the infinite source of love.

WHAT ADVICE DO YOU HAVE FOR CREATING HEALTH AND VITALITY FROM THE INSIDE OUT?

Learn to listen to yourself. Learn to observe. Trust yourself. Trust that everything is just as it should be because life, with all of its twists and turns, is a journey. It is also important that you learn how your body works, because that way you can support it. We live in a world that is not exactly health promoting, so it's important that you are educated. Education will empower you. Knowledge is useless if you don't take action on what you have learned.

It's also super important to ask questions—the really important questions like why things are happening and what is going on. Don't jump to masking symptoms with a pill or a supplement out of fear. That won't give you the results you are seeking. If you want to create health and vitality, you need to have knowledge and you need to trust yourself and your body to know what you need.

Adopt a lifestyle that is similar to our ancestors' because, again, evolution perfected an ecosystem that allows us all to thrive if we allow it to support us. Eat, sleep, exercise, be social, and have a lot of diversity of microbes and foods as well. Let go of a little control and let go of judgment. We always judge something as either good or bad. "I am sick—that's bad" or "I am healthy — therefore it is good." Judgment causes resistance and resistance equals pain and suffering. So, if you can let go of judging and view things as an opportunity to grow and evolve and expand, you'll understand that you are loved no matter what and love is what truly heals.

About the Author

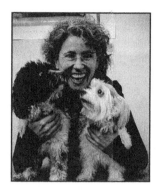

Dr. Odette Suter graduated from veterinary school in Switzerland in 1994. Early on, she recognized the limitations of conventional medicine and questioned its role in true healing. Her healing journey has led her to explore many holistic avenues to uncover and treat the underlying cause of disease of her animal patients.

As a truly holistic vet, she is passionate about education and has written the international best-selling book *What Your Vet Never Told You – Secrets to Supporting Peak Health for Your Animal*. Dr Suter, also lovingly known as Dr. Poop Lady, is a sought-after speaker and teacher in the field of holistic veterinary medicine.

Dr. Suter developed her own training and mentorship program for pet parents and professionals in which she shares her vast experience and knowledge to help empower pet parents in their quest to maximize their animals' health worldwide.

If you are sick and tired of watching your animals suffer and wasting precious time and money, find a mentor who has accomplished what you want to achieve. You will discover the shortcut to go from feeling stuck, frustrated, and in pain because you don't know how to turn your beloved pets' health around to feeling empowered in their care and enjoying a happy, healthy, and joyful life together.

odettesuterdvm.com

Nicole Thibodeau

WHEN AND HOW DID YOU FIRST DISCOVER THE BODY HAS THE INNATE ABILITY TO HEAL ITSELF?

I was initiated to Reiki when I was a young mother. I did Reiki on my son's broken leg, and the doctors were completely amazed by how fast he healed. During that time, I also had migraines and went through burnout. It was difficult and aggravating to deal with that. When I saw the doctors, they would just give me some medications, to which I always had a reaction. I could not understand why the doctors were not able to pinpoint what was going on with me.

I had to turn to someone else to find answers, and that was when I started connecting with the people who did Reiki. They directed me to acupuncture, and the acupuncturist directed me to massage. By working with those healers, I was finally able to reconnect deeply and acknowledge my entire being, not just the physical or the mind. I came to understand both were working together. It is through practicing Reiki with other people that I got a deeper connection to my being and saw how my being was able to heal itself even though I forgot from time to time.

I had a second burnout, but by then I understood what was going on. That helped me to extract myself from the pain and go deeper within my own heart and my own being to tap into that divine wisdom, to tap into healing energy that was already in me. I could give the signal to my body to heal itself and become whole again and not just separate parts.

I had surgery, which caused internal hemorrhaging, and it became clear in that moment that if I panicked, I would not help the doctor who was trying to save my life. That is when I asked Mother Earth to take care of my physical body because I believe deeply we have a connection to the earth and it nurtures our physical body. I gave my spirit over to God/Goddess because I was not able to focus on what I needed to do. I completely trusted that I was being held in divine love and energy. I asked for the doctors to be guided in any action needed to save my life, and that is exactly what happened.

WHY DO YOU THINK IT'S SO IMPORTANT FOR PEOPLE TO BE AWARE OF HOW THE BODY HEALS ITSELF?

It is time for all of us to learn about our own healing power. We are not taught to become sovereign in all aspects of our lives. This complements what modern medicine can do for us, because it's an innate gift or perhaps more of a divine power that we have. It is like a tool kit that we were given at birth, but we never learned how to use.

Some people use it consciously and other people use it unconsciously. That is when they talk a lot about miracles happening. For some people it is important to learn how to use their toolkit consciously. It will open them up to healing on all levels of their being—the physical, mental, emotional, and even on the soul level. Understanding that the body heals itself brings us into wholeness of our divine truth, which creates healing.

It is important to understand that healing comes from within because there are more people and fewer doctors in that reality and living within this world. It is important to know how our body functions and how our body reacts to certain foods, medications, or supplements. Knowing this, we become in sync with nature—with our true nature and with nature itself. We can investigate herbs and many things in nature that can help and heal us. As soon as we become in sync with our whole being and nature, there is no need for an illness or a disease to be in our body.

If it happens, for me, it seems to be unresolved energies that are sitting there. Examining that is the way to clear deeply held belief systems, thoughtforms, and patterns that we hold. That liberates our physical body, which carries those memories. It is time for all of us to free ourselves from debilitating and limiting beliefs, patterns, and thoughtforms.

WHAT ADVICE DO YOU HAVE FOR CREATING HEALTH AND VITALITY FROM THE INSIDE OUT?

Have gratitude for your body working on its own without you having to think about it. Be grateful for its magnificence, its intricacies, and the way it functions every day. Gratitude helps your body receive positive energy, and it is like a boost in energy that you are giving it every time you have gratitude. I have been doing this for years, giving gratitude for my body, even for my stomach if I have a stomach ache. I just thank my stomach for letting me know something is not going well, and I also give thanks to my stomach for functioning so well all of the time.

Always treat your body, mind, and soul as a whole. From working in Reiki, I have seen many people who are desperately ill, and they have not treated themselves wholly. They have separated their body, their mind, their spirit, and their soul. Working as a whole brings healing on a different level. Most of the time your body will stay healed.

You can use healing energy on yourself. If you do not want to learn a modality, then find a healer who resonates with you. Take the time to examine how you resonate with that person. Resonating with your healer helps you release and surrender completely to the process. That means you open yourself completely to reactivate the natural ability of your body to heal itself, giving it the deep message that it is time to reactivate certain parts of your body and certain cells so they can heal.

Find the type of healing that resonates with you as well: acupuncture, massage, sound, energy healing, or Reiki. If you decide to learn these modalities yourself, then perhaps you might be able to help others around you. We all have the keys that will help healing begin.

About the Author

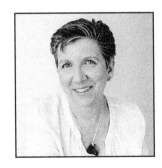

Nicole Thibodeau is a channeler, mentor, and author of *Back to Love Again, A Giver's Guide to Reconnect with Your Inner Strength.*

Nicole supports women who are answering their Soul's calling to open their hearts and connect deeply to their divine self, so they receive more clarity, balance, and harmony in their lives. Using tools, guidance, and a supportive space, she helps them integrate and bring back the higher frequencies of the Divine Blueprint of their Soul and Higher Self.

You can find the Peaceful Heart Principles she uses regularly to recenter and keep herself in a state of Divine Peace at: nicolethibodeau.ca/TIE.

nicolethibodeau.ca
info@nicolethibodeau.ca
IG and FB @nicolethibodeau.ca

Marie-Laure Will

WHEN AND HOW DID YOU FIRST DISCOVER THE BODY HAS THE INNATE ABILITY TO HEAL ITSELF?

I was at Brussels airport in December 2009 getting ready to board a flight to Jerusalem. A team of Israeli Guard policemen mistook me for a terrorist and took me to the basement of the airport for questioning and searches. I asked them, "What's going on?"

Their only answer was, "This is a security procedure."

I felt lost, helpless, and very stressed. They finally released me, and I was able to continue my journey. By the time I arrived in Jerusalem my body was tied in knots.

The next day something surprising happened that would change my life forever. While visiting the Dome of the Ascension on the Mount of Olives, I suddenly had a profound experience of enlightenment. All the stress in my body instantly melted away and a deep peace came over me. My consciousness expanded like an atom in the universe and powerful energetic gifts of healing were activated in me that day.

A few years after, with a perfect management of my gifts, I became Leader #1 of The Quantum Leap as a spiritual healer of rapid transformation.

WHY DO YOU THINK IT'S SO IMPORTANT FOR PEOPLE TO BE AWARE OF HOW THE BODY HEALS ITSELF?

There are five important reasons for people to be aware of how the body heals itself.

1. You need to be aware that your body belongs to you and that you are the only one to hold the ultimate healing power over yourself.

2. The intention, the thought, the energy, the vibration you maintain will determine your level of good health.

3. Illnesses and emotions are the symptoms of old memories buried within you that are waiting to be released to regain alignment and perfect health.

4. To manage your health correctly, you must learn to know your body. Listening to the body is the first step toward healing.

5. A cure without a broad and deep awareness of the origin of the problem is not a cure; it is a

bandage. Eventually you will have to come back to the problem to solve it definitively.

WHAT ADVICE DO YOU HAVE FOR CREATING HEALTH AND VITALITY FROM THE INSIDE OUT?

I agree with Sadhguru's quote: "Without transforming individual human beings, there will be no transformation in the world."

In other words, as long as the human being is not aware of their magic potential buried within, they will constantly put their healing power in the hands of someone else, who will make them believe that they hold the key to the truth of their healing.

Every human being lives in community to grow together. However, we are destined to free ourselves. It is part of our original fundamental nature to access our total autonomy, in our consciousness and in our being, to live free and reveal our great soul in the broad day of humanity.

This is his deepest reason on earth.

About the Author

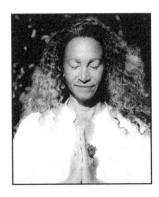

From business woman to spiritual master, Marie-Laure Will's vision is to lead 100 million people to join their Soul Trajectory at the speed of miracle to fulfill who they truly are. The goal? Access to a fulfilling, abundant life, to the self-realization to build a world of compassion and harmony.

Join The Quantum Leap and change your life in twenty-four hours! A unique experience for people who are fearless and determined to create change in their lives.

You can find Marie-Laure Will at: marielaurewill.com

Dr. Liz Winders

WHEN AND HOW DID YOU FIRST DISCOVER THE BODY HAS THE INNATE ABILITY TO HEAL ITSELF?

In 2017, I was on a journey of self-healing after I experienced some medical trauma during the birth of my daughter. During my long journey of healing a medical trauma, I came across a couple of energy healing modalities and felt first-hand the power of landing in a modality that shifts everything and ultimately, changed my entire life.

Subsequently, I learned to sit with pain, whether physical or emotional, and I stopped running from my body. This transformation allowed me to partner with my body in my own self-healing journey. Prior to landing in this wisdom, I had tried all the alternatives. I had gone the traditional route and been disappointed, felt stuck and hopeless, which led to trying out things that I might otherwise not have considered. As I began working with an energy healing modality, I became aware of a greater capacity to be in my body again, to experience joy, to laugh with ease, to settle. It had been four or five years since I had been in that space. That was profound in my state of being. That shifted everything for me. I was more hopeful. I aligned with my purpose. I changed my career and all sorts of positive changes happened for me.

WHY DO YOU THINK IT'S SO IMPORTANT FOR PEOPLE TO BE AWARE OF HOW THE BODY HEALS ITSELF?

Humanity is in a massive time of expansion and evolution. Each one of us has the responsibility to know ourselves, know our wounds, know our ancestral baggage, and to heal ourselves. When we do that, we bring greater light to our own lives, to the lives of our family and friends, to the greater collective, and to the planet. Now is the time to take back our individual power. Looking for external validation or diagnosis or fix or cure has exhausted our individual power. Understanding that brings great wisdom and a powerful capacity within each of us. All healing is self-healing. This wisdom can come from deeply listening to our bodies or from working with a practitioner who honors your experience and knowledge as the most important piece of the healing puzzle.

WHAT ADVICE DO YOU HAVE FOR CREATING HEALTH AND VITALITY FROM THE INSIDE OUT?

Learn to listen to your body's communications with you. We are trained to see an ache or a pain or sadness or other symptoms as bad or wrong. But if you see them as your body giving you an invitation for growth and expansion or giving you the opportunity to know something about yourself, then you can respond to that invitation. Healing happens when you meet the invitation with love and curiosity. Transformation happens in that moment!

You can love and accept what is within your body rather than seeing it as bad or wrong or judging it or denying it. Learn to be with what is in the body. Really listen to your body's communication. Find an expert healer who will walk alongside you on your healing journey and serve as a partner and witness. And finally, give yourself permission for more joy, more pleasure, and less push, less work.

About the Author

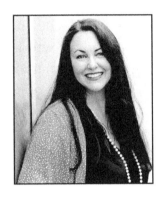

Dr. Liz is a retired clinical psychologist now specializing in Energy Healing and Energetic Coaching. A medical trauma during the birth of her daughter sparked an incredible shift, ultimately aligning her with her soul's purpose. The essence of her work brings clients on a journey from suffering and trauma to empowered and aligned living. She is certified in ten different energy healing modalities that blend beautifully to create a unique healing experience for every client. Dr. Liz lives with her husband and daughter in Durham, North Carolina. In her free time, she enjoys traveling, gardening, and all things with animals and mother nature.

Are you ready to activate your own capacity to self-heal while releasing inner wounds, outdated stories, and trauma? Click here to receive a free download of Dr. Liz's unique Energetic Healing.

essentialhealingwithdrliz.com/welcome

Conclusion

Congratulations on reaching the conclusion of this book. It has been our absolute pleasure to introduce you to these inspirational difference-makers we've featured. It is our hope that you have learned a lot as you read, and that a world of possibilities has opened up for you. Let this not be a book you read once and put down without taking any action.

We highly suggest reading through this book three times and with each read take three action steps toward creating better health and vitality for you, your family, and people that you care about.

Which authors did you connect with most?

Which stories really stuck with you?

Who inspired you the most?

Who made you consider exploring new possibilities that you may not have considered previously?

Which authors do you feel will support you in your current healing journey?

As a next step, we suggest reaching out to them. Make a connection. See how they may support you moving forward.

We wish you all the best in your healing journey.

About the Publisher

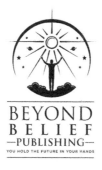

BEYOND
BELIEF
—PUBLISHING—
YOU HOLD THE FUTURE IN YOUR HANDS

In 2004, Babypie Publishing was founded by entrepreneurs Keith and Maura Leon S. when they decided to self-publish their co-authored book, *The Seven Steps to Successful Relationships*. Babypie published its second book, Keith Leon's *Who Do You Think You Are? Discover the Purpose of Your Life* a few years later — implementing a large marketing campaign that introduced the book to over a million people on the first day it came out — and both books became bestsellers overnight.

After the success of their first two titles, Keith and Maura were approached by another author who believed they could take his book to bestseller status as well. They decided to give it a shot, and Warren Henningsen's book *If I Can You Can: Insights of an Average Man* became an international bestseller the day it was released.

Before long, Babypie Publishing was receiving manuscript submissions from all over the world and publishing such titles as Ronny K. Prasad's *Welcome to Your Life*; Melanie Eatherton's *The 7-Minute Mirror*; and Maribel Jimenez and Keith Leon's *The Bake Your Book Program: How to Finish Your Book Fast and Serve It Up HOT!*

With a vision to make an even greater impact, Babypie Publishing began offering comprehensive writing and publishing programs, as well as a full range of à-la-carte services to support independent authors and innovative professionals in getting their message out in the most powerful and effective manner. In 2015, Keith and Maura developed the YouSpeakIt book program to make it easy, fast, and affordable for busy entrepreneurs and cutting-edge health practitioners to get their mission and message out to the world.

In 2016, Leon Smith Publishing was created as the new home for Babypie, YouSpeakIt, and future projects. In 2018, Beyond Belief Publishing was added as an imprint for spiritual and esoteric titles. They have published well over 100 books.

Whether you're a transformational author looking for writing and publishing services or a visionary leader ready to take your life and work to the next level, we thank you for visiting our website at LeonSmithPublishing.com, and we look forward to serving you.

Made in the USA
Monee, IL
05 July 2023

38678274R00116